# FERTILITY-ORIENTED FEMALE REPRODUCTIVE SURGERY

Edited by **Atef Darwish**

**Fertility-oriented Female Reproductive Surgery**
http://dx.doi.org/10.5772/62748
Edited by Atef Darwish

**Contributors**

Roger Hart, Rashi Kalra, Philippe E Dubois, Christophe Dransart, Laurie Putz, Maria-Laura Marotta, Sonja Pop-Trajkovic, Vladimir Antic, Jasmina Popovic, Milan Trenkic, Valeriu Marin Surlin, Stefan Patrascu, Sidonia Maria Saceanu, Anca Patrascu, Hany Lashen, Atef M.M. Darwish

**Published by InTech**

Janeza Trdine 9, 51000 Rijeka, Croatia



**Publishing Process Manager** Maja Bozicevic
**Technical Editor** SPi Global
**Cover** InTech Design team

First published January, 2017
Printed in Croatia

Additional hard copies can be obtained from orders@intechopen.com

Fertility-oriented Female Reproductive Surgery, Edited by Atef Darwish
p. cm.
Print ISBN 978-953-51-2877-9
Online ISBN 978-953-51-2878-6

For EU product safety concerns:
IN TECH d.o.o., Prolaz Marije Krucifikse Kozulić 3, 51000 Rijeka, Croatia,
info@intechopen.com or visit our website at intechopen.com.

# Meet the editor

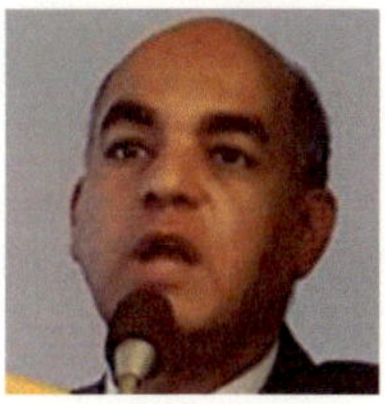

Dr. Atef Darwish graduated from Assiut School of Medicine in 1985 with an excellent grade and first-class honors. He completed a residency in Obstetrics and Gynecology at the Department of Obstetrics and Gynecology, Assiut University and Ain Shams University in 1986–1989. He got his master's degree in 1989 with excellent degree. Between 1992 and 1994, he spent 2 years at the endoscopy unit of Ulm University, Germany. Thereafter, he received his medical doctorate in 1995 through a combined program between the University of Ulm, Germany, and the University of Assiut, Egypt, with excellent degree. He joined many centers in the United States and Europe concentrating on the reproductive medicine. Currently, he is a professor of Obstetrics and Gynecology, Faculty of Medicine, Assiut University since July 2005. Moreover, he is a consultant of Obstetrics and Gynecology in 3 hospitals, and a moderator and lecturer of many endoscopic societies. He authored more than 70 papers and edited 5 books, and presented more than 88 presentations in national and international meetings. His special interest has been in the area of gynecologic laparoscopy and hysteroscopy, reproductive medicine, and assisted reproduction. In 2009, he got a PhD degree in Reproductive Medicine at the University of Utrecht, the Netherlands.

# Contents

# Preface

In modern practice, the role of female reproductive surgery is declining apparently due to the widespread availability of assisted reproductive technology as an attractive option for infertile couples. To be more precise, prevention of female infertility should be the ultimate goal of all obstetricians and gynecologists during operating on females in the reproductive age. Since cesarean section (CS) is the commonest major operation performed on women, the first chapter of this book describes in detail surgical steps required to preserve and enhance future fertility of women subjected to CS. Moreover, remote complications of CS that would jeopardize their future fertility are discussed with clarification of the proper management plan.

Evidence proved that hysteroscopic myomectomy for submucosal fibroids results in higher pregnancy rates. Moreover, hysteroscopic removal of polyps or submucous myomas prior to IUI or ICSI would increase pregnancy rate. In this book, you will read detailed steps of hysteroscopic myomectomy and how to enhance fertility during the procedure. Chapter 2 demonstrates that submucosal fibroids are associated with reduced fertility and an increased miscarriage rate, and if properly treated, the reverse will result.

Endometriosis can compromise fertility in different ways. Surgery would reduce symptoms and improve fertility by removing endometriotic patches, implants, cysts, nodules, and adhesions. Well-designed medical studies clearly showed that destroying even small implants of endometriosis can improve fertility by as much as 50%. Furthermore, monthly pregnancy rate following surgical treatment of minimal, mild, or moderate endometriosis rises. In addition to improving fertility, surgery may often eliminate or improve symptoms of dyspareunia, dysmenorrhea, and pelvic pain, thus improving women's health.

It has been mentioned that you will not diagnose endometriosis unless you are endometriosis-minded. This book contains a full chapter of different methods of diagnosis and proper stratified management plans for pelvic endometriosis (Chapter 3).

Laparoscopy is the gold standard diagnostic as well as therapeutic tool for endometriosis. A separate chapter (Chapter 4) in this book describes in detail laparoscopic techniques to treat endometriosis, even deep infiltrating endometriosis, aiming at fertility preservation.

Not only does laparoscopy improve fertility of endometriosis women, it can also enhance and preserve fertility in other infertile women by performing microsurgical ovarian, tubal, peritoneal, or uterine surgeries. Every effort should be exerted to make laparoscopy a safe and convenient treatment modality. One of the keys of successful laparoscopic surgery is good exposure via a suitable pneumoperitoneum space. In this book, you will read difficulties of exposure of the surgical field during laparoscopy and different methods to overcome including deep neuromuscular blockage technique (Chapter 5).

Advanced pelvic surgery whether performed by laparoscopy or laparotomy may affect pelvic innervations; that is why many endoscopists conceived the concept of nerve-sparing pelvic microsurgery. Whether surgery would affect bowel function or bladder functions is not clearly settled in literature. The last book chapter (Chapter 6) demonstrates the impact of gynecologic operations, particularly hysterectomy on bowel functions in females.

This book has a clear message to all obstetricians and gynecologists. It reminds them that fertility-preservation concept should be put in mind during all surgical procedures. This concept should be extended to cover all pelvic surgeries such as general surgery and urology.

**Atef Darwish, MD, PhD**
Woman's Health University Hospital
Assiut, Egypt

Section 1

# Fertility-oriented Cesarean Section

Chapter 1

# Microsurgical Cesarean Section

Atef Darwish

Additional information is available at the end of the chapter

http://dx.doi.org/10.5772/67123

**Abstract**

Worldwide, not only is cesarean section (CS) the most commonly performed major surgery, but it is also the commonest obstetric operation. CD is associated with some chronic maternal morbidities including pelvic pain, adhesions and adverse reproductive effects. CS carries long-term sequele which can adversely affect subsequent pregnancies. Why do some women develop bad sequele of CS-like adhesions, and infertility is well demonstrated in this chapter. Fertility-oriented step-by-step description of CS techniques is extensively described. Some recent controversial issues related to CS like the development of uterine nitche (isthmocele) at the CS scar site, placenta accrete and the role of cesarean myomectomy are discussed in details. At the end of this chapter, the reader will conceive enjoy fertility-oriented concept of CS.

**Keywords:** cesarean section, fertility, infertility, adhesions, isthmocele, adhesions, cesarean myomectomy

## 1. Introduction

While cesarean section (CS) is sometimes mandatory and even maternal and fetal lifesaving, in most situations, spontaneous vaginal birth is still safer for both woman and her baby. Worldwide, cesarean delivery (CD) is the most frequent major operation performed, and of course, the commonest surgery performed in obstetrics. For instance, in the US, nearly one in three women gives birth by CS. According to The American College of Obstetricians and Gynecologists and the Society for Maternal-Fetal Medicine [1], CD is too common in the US and has markedly increased up to the extent that about 1.3 million children each year are now delivered by CS.

## 2. Epidemiology of CS

Of no doubt, all obstetricians and even the public community notice dramatic increase of CS rate. The rate of CD (calculated by dividing the number of CS over the total number of live births) has increased dramatically since the 1990s, reaching a peak of 32.9% in 2009 [2]. In 1985, the international healthcare community has considered the ideal rate for CS to be between 10 and 15%. Since then, CS has become increasingly performed in both developed and developing countries [3].

In one study [4], the latest CS rates and trends over the last 24 years were presented. According to data from 150 countries, they found that 18.6% of all births occur by CS, ranging from 6 to 27.2% in the least and most developed regions, respectively. Latin America and the Caribbean region had the highest CS rates (40.5%), followed by Northern America (32.3%), Oceania (31.1%), Europe (25%), Asia (19.2%) and Africa (7.3%). It was concluded that the use of CS worldwide has increased to unprecedented levels although the gap between higher- and lower-resource settings remains. Practically speaking, CS rates show every day increase thanks to improved safety issues, refinement of the surgical techniques and maternal preference.

The increased rate of CS can be seen among women of all ages and race/ethnicities, in every country, and across all gestational ages. Because the primary CD rate has increased and the rate of trial of labor after CD has decreased, the primary CS rate has become a major driver in the total CD rate. Moreover, contributing to the high CD rate is increased subjective indications, for example, fetal distress or nonreassuring fetal heart rate (FHR) tracing and failure of progress in addition to elective CS [2].

### 2.1. CS and female fertility

A lot of women subjected to CD can easily get pregnant even within 2 months after the operation. There is a general consensus among obstetricians and women that CS has little compromise of future fertility. Unfortunately, this consensus is not based on respectable studies. Personal impression or experience even of scientific committees is class IV evidence.

### 2.2. Why CS is less likely to induce pelvic adhesions compared to gynecologic operations?

Regarding the risk of fertility-related adhesions, the nearer the surgery to the pelvis, the higher risk of adhesion formation. Any gynecologic or nongynecologic pelvic surgery is considered as a potential risk factor for pelvic adhesion induction.

Nevertheless, adhesion formation after CS is less likely than gynecologic operations which may be attributed to one or more of the following [5]:

- Less tissue hypoxia due to greater tissue perfusion associated with physiological changes in pregnancy.
- The injured site at rest: the lower segment (LS) is subjected to fewer movements than upper segment (US). LSCS site is the least susceptible site for adhesion formation. That is why

we recommend performing myomectomy of the anterior uterine wall or even some fundal myomata via a LSCS-like incision to minimize adhesion formation. The same concept applies for cervical myoma after proper dissection of the bladder.

- LS is covered by UB which is constantly being filled and emptied during the healing process disrupting any fibrinous band between the uterus and the bladder, and between the LS and the anterior abdominal wall, thus decreasing adhesion development at this location.
- Anatomic effects of uterine involution postpartum would help disruption of newly formed adhesions.
- Always single incision (unlike myomectomy where more than one incision may be required).
- Rare hematoma formation.

*2.2.1. Minimal adhesion risk peculiar to pregnancy*

- Pregnancy is associated with increased fibrinolytic activity in amniotic fluid beyond 37 weeks.
- During pregnancy, there is increased plasminogen activator activity which is associated with fewer adhesion formation risks.
- Unique hormonal changes of pregnancy with increased steroid section.

*2.2.2. Clinical evidence of lower adhesion formation rate following CS*

Since CD incision is away from the tubes and hidden by the bladder flap, it is expected to develop fewer adhesions than posterior or fundal uterine incisions [6]. A second-look laparoscopy assessed adhesions between the abdominal wall and the underlying omentum and bowel following a previous laparotomy [7]. Patients with midline incisions performed for gynecologic indications had significantly more adhesions than all types of incisions performed for obstetric indications (OR, 1.65; CI, 0.97–2.83, $P = .054$). The presence of adhesions in patients with previous obstetric surgery was not affected by the type of incision in this study. Similarly, women with midline or Pfannenstiel incision for gynecologic surgery had more adhesions than those with incisions for obstetric surgery [8].

However, adhesions continue to occur despite lower uterine incisions, albeit less to the anterior abdominal wall compared to classical upper segment CD or gynecologic incisions.

### 2.3. Deleterious impact of CS on subsequent fertility

Sometimes, CD is associated with some chronic maternal morbidities including pelvic pain, adhesions and adverse reproductive effects like decreased fertility and increased risk of spontaneous abortion and ectopic pregnancy [9]. Pelvic adhesions may cause pelvic pain, dyspareunia, intestinal obstruction or infertility. CS carries long-term sequele which can adversely affect subsequent pregnancies. Women with previous CS may present with frequent intermenstrual spotting due to retention of blood inside a reservoir-like defect of the scar (isthmocele). Generally, women who have had a CS are less likely to have further children than those who have had a vaginal delivery. This can be attributed to voluntary family planning, patient fear from repeated surgical intervention, consequences of the indications for the cesarean and due to the operation itself.

On evaluation of 18 cohort studies [10], it has been found the CS is associated with **9%** reduction of subsequent pregnancy rate [risk ratio (RR) 0.91, 95% confidence interval (CI) (0.87, 0.95)] and **11%** reduction of birth rate [RR 0.89, 95%CI (0.87, 0.92)] compared with patients who had delivered vaginally.

However, these studies were heterogeneous with failure to assess some contributing factors like increasing maternal age (which is the most important independent fertility factor), changes in accepted indications for elective CS and changes in women's choices (increased CS on demand rate). **CS on demand (maternal request) is** primary prelabor CS on maternal request in the absence of any maternal or fetal indications.

### 2.4. How does CS induce adhesions?

Surgery may cause tissue ischemia which is a predisposing factor for adhesion formation. Subsequently, suppression of fibrinolysis and persistence of fibrin follow. Immunosuppression may have a role. Additive rough surgical techniques would aggravate adhesion formation like aggressive tissue manipulations, use of excessive electrocoagulation, leaving FB particles or blood during surgery, infection and any factor damaging the normal healing process [11].

#### *2.4.1. Impact of post-CD adhesions on the operative course of repeat CS*

All obstetricians face some difficulties with variable degrees due to adhesions induced by a previous CD. The incidence of adhesion development increases with the number of CDs performed. A significantly higher risk of intraperitoneal adhesions was detected in patients undergoing their 4th to 10th CD compared to those having their 1st, 2nd or 3rd CD (OR, 8.1; CI, 2.7–23.8) [12]. One study [13] was constructed to estimate the incidence of adhesions after CS and to determine their impact on delivery and infant well-being.

They evaluated reports of 542 women who had undergone primary CS (265 women) or repeat CS (277 women). The incidence, severity, and locations of adhesions, delivery time, cord blood pH, and Apgar scores were analyzed. After the first CD, 100 of 217 women (46%) had pelvic adhesive disease; 48 of 64 women (75%) who underwent a third CD and 5 of 6 women (83%) who underwent a fourth CD had formed pelvic adhesive disease. Compared with primary CD, delivery of the infant was delayed 5.6 min (52%) with 1 previous CD, 8.5 min (79%) after 2 CD, and 18.1 min (169%) during the fourth CD ($P < 0.001$ for all comparisons).It had been concluded that the high percentage of CDs results in adhesive disease, which delays repeat CD of the fetus. The potential for adhesive disease should be included in counseling regarding primary elective CD. Actually, I find the last conclusion very valuable as women are not familiar with long-term sequele of CD particularly surgical difficulties and possibility of additional surgical procedures like adhesiolysis, repair of bladder injury or surgical steps required for prompt management of placenta accreta which may end by cesarean hysterectomy.

### 2.5. Impact of CD on the endometrium

CD induces a delay in endometrial maturation at the scar site which might have been a result of disruption in steroid receptor expression, leading to abnormal response to estrogen and progesterone [14]. Endometrium at LSCS scar site may not cycle in synchrony with the rest of endometrium in the uterine cavity. Endometrial samples were taken from both cesarean scar site and posterior uterine wall and were compared to similar samples obtained from women who had spontaneous vaginal delivery (SVD). Fewer leukocytes and less vascularization at the scar site were seen less than in the endometrium of the unscarred uterus.

### 2.6. Other CD-associated abnormal uterine factors

CD may be associated with abnormal scar healing, abnormal signaling, disturbed endometrial receptivity as well as uterine contractility.

### 2.7. How does CS affect future fertility?

CS can affect fertility by different ways. Principally, CS can cause fertility-compromising induction of intraperitoneal or intrauterine adhesions. Formation of adhesions is common after cesarean delivery; rates of 11–70% have been reported [15].

### 2.8. Possible sites of adhesions following CS

Post-CS adhesions can be seen at different parts of the pelvis and abdomen. Commonly, we notice a thick central band attracting the uterus upward to the anterior abdominal wall as seen by laparoscopy (**Figure 1**). The exact mechanism of formation of this thick band can be attributed to leaving row sites of the scar that adhere to the peritoneum particularly if nonclosure technique is used. This position is fertility-compromising as both tubes will be elevated and fimbriae will not reach the pouch of Douglas for ovum pick-up. In many cases, despite no adhesion detection in the pouch of Douglas at laparoscopy, yet infertility is supposed to be due to abnormal position of the tubes.

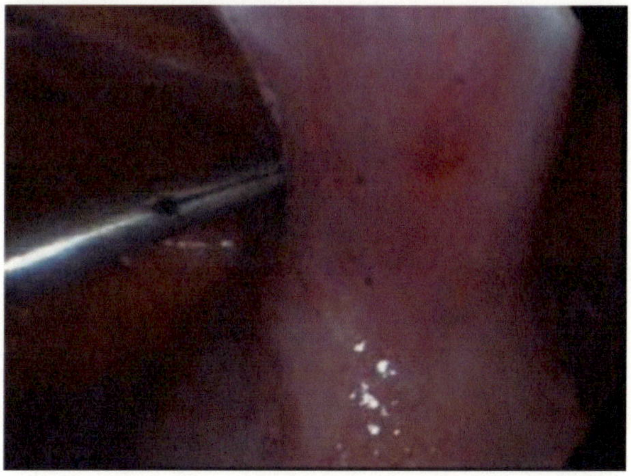

**Figure 1.** A thick central band of post-CS adhesions.

Another commonly seen form of adhesions is lateral position of one or both adnexae with dense adhesions to the lateral pelvic wall (**Figure 2**) or even anterior abdominal wall. These adhesions entrap the ovum and hinder the motility of the tube. Occurrence of such adhesions can be attributed to leaving blood clots or meconium behind in flanks or using dry towels in flanks. The last procedure is practiced by many obstetricians aiming at prevention of soiling the peritoneal cavity with blood, meconium, amniotic fluid or debris. However, serosal trauma induced by towels especially dry towels would be more harmful to the patient from fertility point of view. A very rare but very serious complication of inserting tools in flanks is missing one or both towels which had been seen at least once by some senior obstetricians.

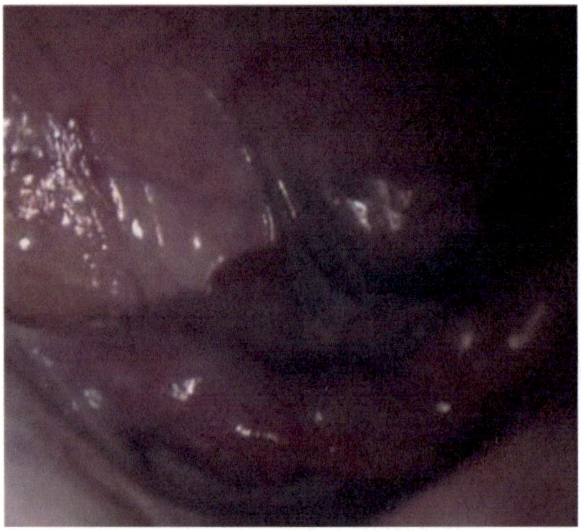

**Figure 2.** Dense adnexal adhesions to lateral pelvic wall.

We may diagnose dense omental (**Figure 3**) and even intestinal adhesions to the anterior abdominal wall, uterovesical pouch, or adnexae. These forms of adhesions result from peritoneal soiling, uterine exterioration or rough manipulations of pelvic organs or intestine.

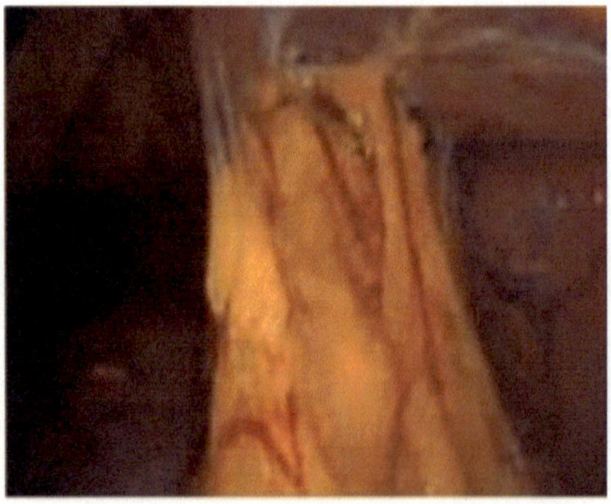

**Figure 3.** Dense omental adhesions.

Fine thin adhesions of the pouch of Douglas (**Figure 4**) can be noticed due to retained blood clots. Excision of these filmy adhesions would increase the chance of pregnancy by facilitating easy ovum pickup.

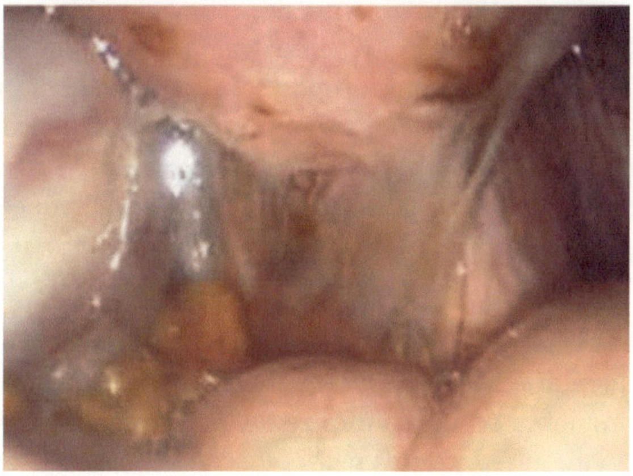

**Figure 4.** Fine adhesions of the pouch of Douglas.

Adhesions can occur in utero. The most difficult and aggressive form of adhesions is class IV intrauterine adhesions (IUAs) (**Figure 5**), which may result from suturing of the anterior and posterior uterine walls, leaving intrauterine remnants (part of placenta or membranous tissues) or post-CS intrauterine infection.

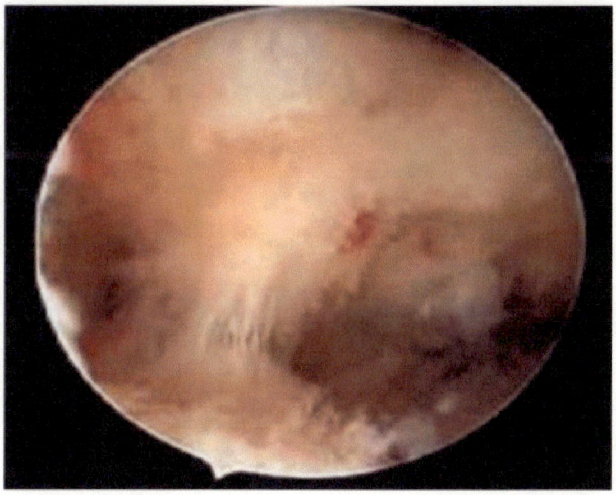

**Figure 5.** Dense IUAs.

### 2.9. Steps of fertility-oriented CS

Some procedures related to CS would affect future fertility including preoperative, intraoperative and postoperative issues. In the following section, stress on impact of every CS step on future fertility will be addressed.

### *2.9.1. Strict asepsis*

The concept of asepsis all through CS should be conceived by all members of the team concerned in delivery process. Every now and then, senior obstetricians should check steps of asepsis by different members of the delivery team. They should inform juniors and nurses that infection is a real enemy to delivery whether vaginal or abdominal. They should teach juniors that washing hands even with antiseptic solutions is not sterilization. Principles of hand cleaning, disinfection and sterilization should be highlighted all the time. Scrubbing hands and forearms even with antiseptic solutions make them "surgically clean." The purpose of scrubbing is to minimize the possibility of infection whenever unintentional cut of sterile gloves occurs and to minimize the risk of infecting the surgeon himself. Senior should check how the team wears gloves and gowns without touching the external surfaces.

Preoperatively, repeated vaginal examination may carry a risk of introduction of ascending infection to the upper genital tract with subsequent fertility compromise. I think that routine use of partograph during labor would minimize the need for repeated vaginal examination. Of course, if PV is highly required, complete aseptic conditions are mandatory.

Some obstetricians routinely clean the vagina with an antiseptic solution which looks a good safety step to guard against ascending infection. Preoperative vaginal cleansing with povidone iodine has reduced post-cesarean infectious morbidities [16].

Prolonged premature rupture of fetal membranes (PROM) is an important factor that would increase the risk of upper genital tract infections and subsequent fertility compromise.

If CS is decided, proper skin disinfection from the lower border of the breasts to the knees is mandatory. Sterilization should be unidirectional using copious amount of the disinfectant. The incision site should be repeatedly disinfected. Whether to use povidone-iodine or chlorhexidine-alcohol is equally effective [17].

**Prophylactic antibiotics:** pre-skin IV BS antibiotic would help reduce maternal infectious morbidity [18].

### *2.9.2. Fertility-oriented skin incision*

Vertical incision allows good access to the pelvis, lower and upper abdomen. However, in addition to being noncosmetic and not accepted by many women, it may affect future fertility. It may attract more adhesions due to longer row space of the peritoneum putting in mind that the row peritoneal surface is not masked unlike transverse incision. The uterus can easily adhere to the peritoneal defect that causes a commonly seen thick central band of adhesions attracting the uterus upward. If the patient became infertile, laparoscopic access to the abdomen will be more dangerous than transverse incision with a possibility of intestinal adhesions to the peritoneal surface. So, it is better to perform transverse incision whenever possible.

Two common transverse incisions for cesarean delivery are performed [6]. The Pfannenstiel skin incision is slightly curved, 2–3 cm above the symphysis pubis, with the midportion of the incision within the shaved area of the pubic hair. The Joel-Cohen type incision is straight, 3 cm below the line that joins the anterior superior iliac spines, and slightly more cephalad than Pfannenstiel [19]. The former incision is usually completed utilizing sharp dissection while the latter using blunt dissection. In a Cochrane meta-analyses of randomized trials of surgical incisions for cesarean delivery, the Joel-Cohen type incision had significant short-term advantages compared with the Pfannenstiel incision, including lower rates of fever, postoperative pain, and use of analgesia, less blood loss and shorter operating time (overall and incision-to-delivery) and hospital stay [20, 21]. In two trials (411 women) that compared the Joel-Cohen incision with the Pfannenstiel incision, the Joel-Cohen incision resulted in a 65% reduction in reported postoperative febrile morbidity (RR 0.35, 95% CI 0.14–0.87); one trial reported reduced postoperative analgesic requirements (RR 0.55, 95% CI 0.40–0.76), operating time (mean difference [MD] -11.40, 95% CI -16.55 to -6.25 min), delivery time (MD -1.90, 95% CI -2.53 to -1.27 min), total dose of analgesia in the first 24 h (MD -0.89, 95% CI -1.19 to -0.59), estimated blood loss (MD -58.00, 95% CI -108.51 to -7.49 mL), postoperative hospital stay for the mother (MD -1.50, 95% CI -2.16 to -0.84 days), and increased time to the first dose of analgesia (MD 0.80, 95% CI 0.12–1.48 h) [20]. No other significant differences were found in either trial.

From fertility-enhancing point of view, transverse incisions are more fertility-enhancing due to direct access to the lower segment with minimal manipulations of the genital organs. Moreover, sutures are confined to the lower segment of the anterior aspect of the uterus away from the adnexae.

#### 2.9.3. *Opening the peritoneum*

It seems that both sharp and blunt opening of the peritoneum have little impact on fertility. Despite no supportive studies on the effect of peritoneal opening on fertility, blunt opening minimizes the risk of inadvertent injury to bowel, bladder or other organs that may be adherent to the underlying surface. This peculiar advantage avoids extra procedures and suturing which may compromise subsequent fertility.

An extraperitoneal approach is another option. Most obstetricians are not familiar with this technique since it was used primarily in the pre-antibiotic era to decrease the risk of intraperitoneal infection. It requires a detailed knowledge of the relationship between the fascial planes the bladder and lower uterine segment. Theoretically, avoiding exposure of the peritoneal cavity to blood, amniotic fluid, vernix, and mechanical irritation can potentially reduce nausea and vomiting, postoperative pain, voiding disturbances, and other side effects and complications of cesarean delivery [6]. This hypothesis is supported by a small randomized trial that compared the transperitoneal and extraperitoneal techniques and found the latter resulted in less intraoperative nausea and vomiting and less postoperative pain [22].

#### 2.9.4. *Prior dense intraperitoneal adhesions*

If there are dense adhesions between the anterior abdominal wall and the anterior surface of the uterus, please enter the peritoneum as lateral as possible bluntly and as close as possible to the upper abdomen to avoid areas of dense scar tissue in the lower abdomen (pelvis). Sharp dissection of the peritoneum also may be needed and should be performed cautiously using shallow incisions under direct vision. If pelvic adhesions are dense and organs are sealed, bladder injury would be inevitable. In such situation, a higher hysterotomy incision albeit more bloody would be obligatory. After delivery of the baby, uterine exterioration may be needed to perform proper adhesiolysis and meticulous hemostasis.

#### *2.9.5. Bladder flap*

It is not clearly cited whether undergoing or omitting development of a bladder flap would affect future fertility. Omitting this procedure reduced the incision-to-delivery interval by an average of one to two minutes and was not associated with an increase in adverse short-term outcome [23, 24]. However, there is no available data to definitively assess morbidity, such risk of bladder injury, or the long-term consequences of not creating a bladder flap.

#### *2.9.6. Fertility-oriented hysterotomy incision*

Of no doubt, transverse incision along the lower uterine segment (i.e., Monro Kerr or Kerr incision) is much more fertility-enhancing than longitudinal incision in different ways including less subsequent adhesion formation, stronger scar with less liability to weakness complications, and less bloody. The problem of the transverse incision is failure to extract the presenting part easily particularly if it is big or the lower segment is not well formed. In such cases, wound extension with subsequent uterine arteries tear is expected. This would require additional rescue procedures that may compromise fertility by induction of adhesions due to excessive bleeding or additional suturing.

A practical trick to minimize the possibility of uterine artery injury is widening of the hysterotomy incision by simultaneous cephalad and caudal traction of the edges using two fingers on the upper and two fingers on the lower end. Never extend the incision right and left as vessel injury would be expected. However, if the presenting part is still not easily extracted, a modification of the wound would be a rescue additional step by doing unilateral or even bilateral curved incisions (J-shaped or U-shaped incisions) with care not to cut the uterine arteries.

Do not perform inverted T-shaped incision whenever possible as it is an agley scar with poor healing and subsequent high possibility of uterine rupture in subsequent pregnancy. In all situations, transverse hysterotomy incision is much better than low vertical or classical vertical incisions simply due to less liability of adhesion formation or compromise the course of subsequent pregnancy.

#### *2.9.7. Exteriorizing the uterus*

It allows more access to the hysterotomy site and adnexae. However, it encourages the surgeon to overmanipulate adnexae with prolonged exposure, congestion and dryness. These factors would increase the possibility of adhesion formation.

A meta-analysis of randomized trials of extraabdominal (exteriorized) versus intraabdominal (in situ) repair found no clinically significant differences in blood loss, intraoperative nausea, vomiting or pain between the two approaches [25]. Unfortunately, it was a short-term study and missed evaluation of future fertility.

### *2.9.8. Finger or instrumental dilatation of cervix*

It aims to improve drainage of blood and lochia. Personally, I routinely perform cervical dilatation in elective CS particularly primigravida where the cervix is tightly closed. We noticed that omission of this step is associated with frequent women complaints of no or trivial vaginal bleeding, and they consider all postoperative complaints due to retained blood inside the uterine cavity. However, risk of ascending infection from the cervix should be considered. The surgeon should change his gloves or discard the used curved artery forceps after cervical dilatation. So far, there are no bacteriological studies on bacterial colonies on the forceps or the gloves after dilatation.

### *2.9.9. Fertility-oriented hysterotomy suturing*

**Choice of suture material:** A plethora of suturing materials is available like chromic catgut or delayed absorbable synthetic, for example, polyglactin 910, poliglecaprone 25. We commonly use 0-delayed absorbable synthetic monofilament (e.g., Monocryl) or braided (e.g., Vicryl) in modern practice. Despite no available studies on the direct relation of suturing material to future fertility, yet we have to select the least tissue-irritant material with minimal tissue reaction.

**Myometrial closure**: Several studies compared single- versus double-layer closure of hysterotomy incision. For fertility enhancement, we usually perform a two-layer, continuous closure with delayed absorbable synthetic suture incorporating all of the muscle to avoid bleeding from the incision edges. Care should be considered to avoid leaving row surface of the scar which is a potential site for further adhesion formation.

**Endometrial suturing**: Previously, it was recommended that the endometrium should be spared from suturing for fear of induction of intrauterine synechiae. However, with frequent sonographic follow-up, it was found that better to include the endometrial layer in the full thickness myometrial closure to avoid scar defect. This opinion is based on a randomized trial that assigned 78 term pregnant patients delivered by cesarean to one layer myometrial closure either including or excluding the endometrial layer [26]. The frequency of a wedge-type healing defect on ultrasound 6 weeks postpartum (isthmocele) was significantly lower in the group that had full thickness suturing (45 versus 69%). It is conceived that isthmocele would negatively affect future fertility (see section on isthmocele and fertility).

**Blunt (rounded tip) versus sharp (tapered point) needles:** Despite performing faster particularly in repeat CS, sharp needles are associated with minute bleeding after traction on the continuous sutures with a possibility of diathermy use. Theoretically, this would increase the likelihood of adhesion invitation. There are no available studies on adhesion formation according to the type of needle so far.

**Single- versus double-layer closure**: It is a controversial issue. From fertility point of view, better to do meticulous two layers without leaving row points. If fertility future is not important, the obstetrician is free to do single- or double-layer closure according to the myometrial thickness and control of bleeding. In a 2014 systematic review and meta-analysis of comparative studies, single- and double-layer hysterotomy closure resulted in similar rates of overall maternal infectious morbidity, endometritis, wound infection, and blood transfusion, but operative time was 6 min shorter with the single-layer closure (20 studies including almost 15,000 patients) [27]. Over the long term, however, uterine rupture in the next pregnancy is a potential risk of single-layer closure [6]. Available data are limited and do not provide convincing evidence of safety or harm. In the 2014 meta-analysis described above, single-layer closure resulted in a nonstatistical increase in "uterine rupture or dehiscence" in the next pregnancy (4.8 versus 2.9%; RR 2.38, 95% CI 0.63–8.96; two studies, n = 187 participants) [27]. The technique used for the single-layer closure may be a contributing factor. Compared with an unlocked closure, locked closure has been associated with higher occurrence of surrogate markers of scar weakness (thinner myometrial thickness, bell-shaped uterine wall defects) [28, 29] and dehiscence or rupture [30]. However, available data are limited by heterogeneity in criteria for diagnosis of uterine scar defects, length of follow-up, method of follow-up, and closure technique, as well as lack of randomization for the primary outcome and the low number of uterine ruptures. Further study of possible adverse consequences of single-layer closure is warranted [6].

**Peritoneal closure and future fertility:** Nonclosure of the visceral or parietal peritoneum saves time with rare liability to postoperative ilius.

Theoretically, nonclosure might allow the enlarged uterus to adhere to the anterior abdominal wall or impede spontaneous closure of the peritoneum, while closure might cause a foreign body reaction to sutures and tissue damage [6].

A systematic review of prospective observational studies of peritoneal nonclosure at CS, nonclosure was associated with greater adhesion formation than closure of the parietal layer or both visceral and parietal layers (OR 2.6, 95% CI 1.48–4.56; three studies, n = 249) [31]. Moreover, a 2011 systematic review that included many of the excluded observational studies in the systematic review [32] also found that nonclosure was associated with greater adhesion formation [33]. On the other hand, some studies found that closure or nonclosure of the peritoneum at CS did not lead to large differences in the adhesion rate [31] using adhesion scoring system.

**Use of drains**: Despite not recommended by many studies, again if the obstetrician is fertility-oriented, intraperitoneal or subrectal tube drains may have a role particularly in repeat cases with concomitant adhesiolysis, ovarian cystectomy or myomectomy. Drain is of peculiar importance if the surgeon closes the abdomen on trivial serosal oozing. In a 2013 meta-analysis of randomized trials of wound drainage at cesarean delivery, routine use of wound drains was not beneficial [34]. Compared with no drain, routine use of drains does not reduce the odds of seroma, hematoma, infection or wound disruption. Additionally, restricted use of subrectus sheath drains offers no benefit in maternal infectious morbidity compared with liberal use [35]. These findings also apply to obese women [36]. All these studies omitted evaluation of further fertility particularly in repeat cases and didn't include laparoscopic findings in infertile cases.

### 2.10. Postpartum care and future fertility

It seems logic that a woman delivered by abdominal approach is more liable to infection than those delivered vaginally. This can be attributed to tissue manipulations, hematoma formation, seroma formation, or leaving behind intraperitoneal blood, AF, meconium or vernix. All these contributing factors are actually added to possible risk factors after vaginal delivery that may help introduce infection to the upper genital tract with subsequent adhesion formation. An additional risk factor is wound infection which may be aggressive to the extent of necrotizing fasciitis. Prompt and condensed treatment of these factors would minimize the risk of adhesion formation.

### 2.11. Bad surgical technique and nonmicrosurgical approach: how to avoid?

- **Think fertility:** To perform microsurgical CS, the surgeon should think fertility all the time. He has to develop the skill of fine manipulations and gentle tissue handling aiming at preservation of future fertility potential of the genital organs. Every effort should be exerted to avoid development of postoperative adhesions which would affect future fertility. Surgeons should adopt a routine adhesion reduction strategy with good surgical practice to reduce adhesion formation [37].
- **Avoid predisposing factors for adhesion formation:** Many factors can contribute for adhesion formations like excessive tissue ischemia, dryness of surfaces, excessive suturing, omental patches or infection. Moreover, technical problems may help adhesions like excessive traction on the peritoneum, retained blood clots inside the peritoneal cavity, prolonged operative time, and adnexal trauma by rough manipulations, dry towels or talc powder. Of peculiar occurrence during CD, leaving meconium and amniotic fluid behind particularly in the Douglas pouch and flanks represents an evident factor as these foreign materials may induce peritoneal and serosal irritation with subsequent inflammation.
- **Microsurgical principles:** An obstetrician should think microsurgery during CS. He should follow fertility-preserving reconstructive surgical principles which are as follows:
- Avoidance of serosal insults: tissue trauma, ischemia, hemorrhage, infection, foreign-body reaction, and leaving raw surfaces.
- Minimizing tissue trauma by using atruamatic techniques, meticulous hemostasis, complete excision of abnormal tissues and precise alignment and approximation of tissue planes. Since a long time, there is some evidence of superiority of reconstructive surgery over nonreconstructive surgery. For instance, performing reconstructive surgical correction of distal tubal occlusion achieved double pregnancy rate if compared to nonreconstructive technique surgical [38].

### 2.12. Safety guidelines against adhesion formation during CS

Despite principally described for gynecologic operations [39], most of the following six safety guidelines (with some modifications to suite CS) can properly apply for CS.

1. The risk of postoperative adhesions should be systematically discussed with any patient scheduled for open or laparoscopic abdominal surgery prior to obtaining his/her informed consent.
2. Surgeons need to act to reduce postoperative adhesions in order to fulfill their duty of care toward patients undergoing abdominal surgery.
3. Surgeons should adopt a routine adhesion reduction strategy (especially for women more prone liable to adhesions like those with prolonged PROM, or those with a history of postoperative adhesions or laparoscopic adhesiolysis due to previous CS).
4. Good surgical technique is fundamental to any adhesion reduction strategy.
   a. Carefully handle tissue with field enhancement (magnification) techniques (in CS good illumination is sufficient).
   b. Focus on planned surgery and, if any secondary pathology is identified, question the risk: benefit ratio of surgical treatment before proceeding (like performing cesarean myomectomy or ovarian cystectomy during CS).
   c. Perform diligent hemostasis and ensure diligent use of cautery (better bipolar with minimal secondary coagulation effect).
   d. Reduce diathermy time and frequency and aspirate aerosolized tissue following diathermy.
   e. Excise tissue—reduce fulguration.
   f. Reduce duration of surgery (whenever possible to minimize tissue dryness).
   g. Reduce risk of infection.
   h. Reduce drying of tissues.
   i. Limit use of sutures and choose fine nonreactive sutures.
   j. Avoid foreign bodies when possible—such as materials with loose fibers.
   k. Avoid nonperitonized implants and meshes.
   l. Minimal use of dry towels or sponges in laparotomy.
   m. Use starch- and latex-free gloves in laparotomy.
5. Surgeons should consider the use of adhesion reduction agents as part of the adhesion reduction strategy.
   i. Give special consideration to agents with data supporting safety in routine surgery and efficacy in adhesion prevention
   ii. Practicality, ease of use, and cost of agents should influence their selection for routine practice

iii. Good medical practice implies that any serious or frequently occurring risks be discussed before obtaining the patient's informed consent prior to surgery.

### 2.13. How to fight against infertility induced by CD?

#### *2.13.1. Increase patient and doctor awareness about fertility compromising sequele of CS*

**Back to normal delivery:** Obstetricians should be very clear when counseling women for CS. We should emphasize that CS is a major operation with a lot of complications up to maternal death. Counseling regarding future fertility should include studies which documented decreased pregnancy rate after CS especially repeat CS. The risk of placenta accreta and the possibility of hysterectomy in subsequent pregnancies should be addressed.

**Discourage CS on demand and unnecessary CD:** A good number of CS is done in situations when babies could be safely delivered vaginally instead. Sometimes, performing CS when it is not necessary poses avoidable risks to the mother and her child and needlessly raises costs, research shows [40].

Potential risks of CS on maternal request include a longer maternal hospital stay, an increased risk of respiratory problems for the infant, and greater complications in subsequent pregnancies, including uterine rupture, placental implantation problems, and the need for hysterectomy. Potential short-term benefits of planned CS compared with a planned vaginal delivery which may end in selective CS include a decreased risk of hemorrhage and transfusion, fewer surgical complications, and a decrease in urinary incontinence during the first year after delivery. CS on maternal request particularly is not recommended for women desiring several children, given that the risks of placenta previa, placenta accreta, and gravid hysterectomy increase with each CS [40].

#### *2.13.2. Endoscopic (laparoscopic and hysteroscopic) management of CS-induced infertility*

**(A) Laparoscopic uterolysis (Figure 6):** Thick central band between the uterus and the anterior abdominal wall can be expected on clinical examination where the cervix is high or inaccessible at all in addition to restricted mobility on vaginal examination. At laparoscopy, the uterus may be seen densely adherent and attracted to the anterior abdominal wall. In some cases, we found the uterus very near to the umbilicus. After proper evaluation of the pelvis and sometimes extensive adhesiolysis of omental adhesions, access to the uterovesical pouch is confirmed. If the cervix is vaginally accessible even with some traction, the assistant should insert a uterine manipulator to push on aiming at finding a space for work. Trial of uterolysis should start by cutting the thick central band of adhesions using a scissors or a microneedle which will help lateral dissection. In the same time, lateral counter pressure on the uterus should be done by a blunt instrument to facilitate adhesiolysis. Sometimes, this band is thin but may not be identifiable due to sealing of the uterus in the anterior abdominal wall. In such cases, using a microneedle, sharp dissection of the uterus is done with control of bleeding points using a coagulating probe.

Care should be taken whenever the base of the band is reached to avoid bladder injury. Of good clinical importance is the frequent insertion of a metal catheter into the bladder to ensure intact wall. Lysis should be stopped after completion of uterine freeing and easy access to the cervix vaginally. Secure hemostasis and peritoneal toilet are essential.

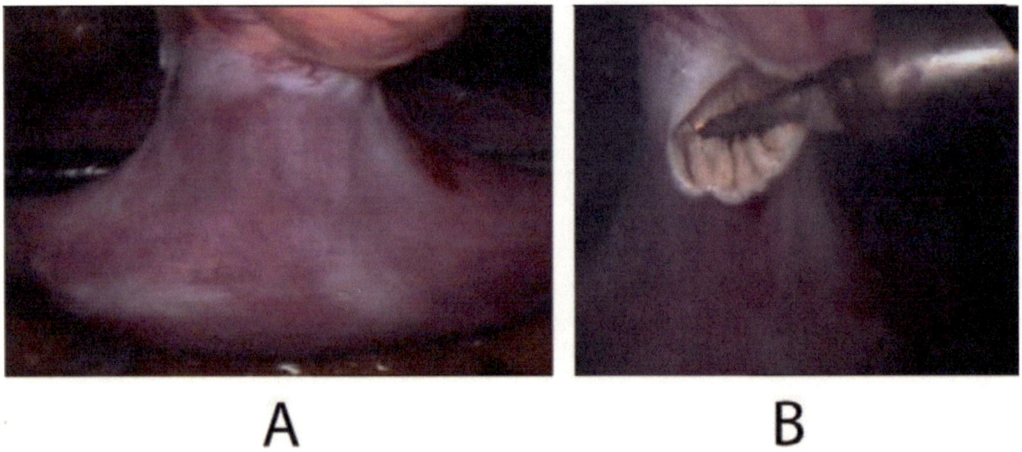

**Figure 6.** Adhesiolysis of the central thick band: (A) before cutting and (B) during cutting.

**(B) Laparoscopic adnexolysis:** Sometimes, the adnexa are densely adherent to the lateral pelvic wall (**Figure 7**). Firstly, the relationship of the adnexa to the vital iliac vessels should be identified. Unlike uterolysis, dissection would rely mainly on blunt dissection and counter traction to avoid vessel injury. If sharp dissection is required, it should be done ontracted adnexa to the other side and the tips of the scissors directed medially toward the adnexa.

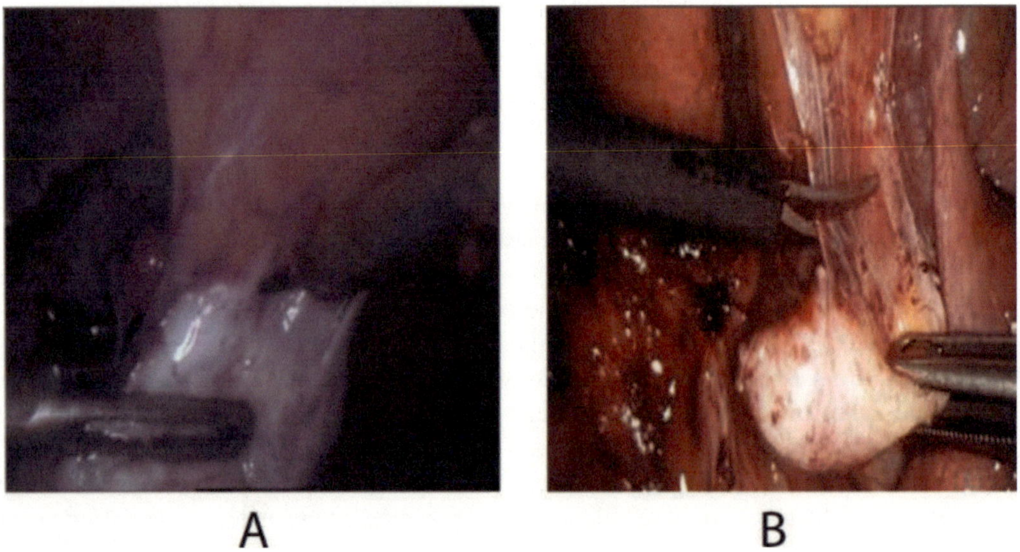

**Figure 7.** Adnexolysis: (A) counter traction to the opposite side and (B) cutting against attracted adnexa.

**(C) Microsurgical adhesiolysis** of any other fertility-related adhesions is usually done using a sharp scissors (**Figure 8**).

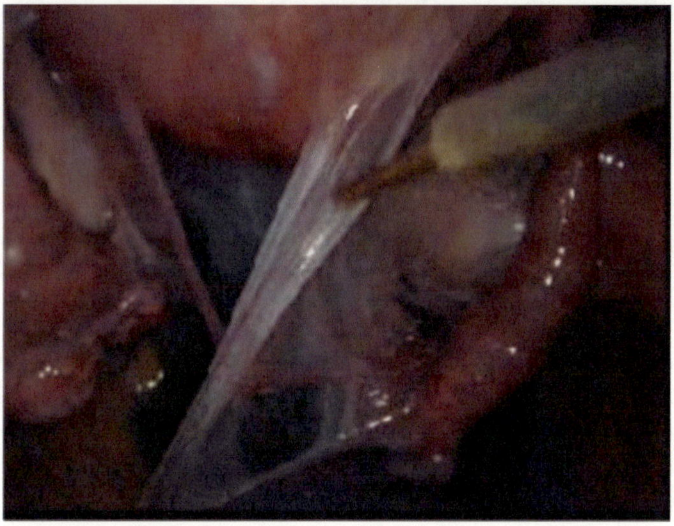

**Figure 8.** Adhesiolysis.

**(D) Hysteroscopic adhesiolysis (HA)** essentially should be preceded by grading of adhesions either by hysterosalpingography or better by office hysteroscopy. The hysteroscopist plans the procedure according to the grade. Sometimes more than one session is required. Different tools can be used according to the availability and expertise. A 5-mm office operative hysteroscopy or the standard 9-mm conventional hysteroscope may be used (**Figure 9**). Flexible or rigid scissor can be used by experienced hyseroscopists (**Figure 9**). Bipolar electrode is a good option for adhesiolysis as well. The main goal of adhesiolysis is to restore a uterine cavity suitable for implantation and maintenance of normal pregnancy. Postoperative intrauterine balloon left for 1–2 weeks or IUCD left for 1 month may be required to avoid reformation of adhesions. A postoperative course of estrogens would be required to enhance growth of the normal endometrium to cover areas previously occupied by adhesions.

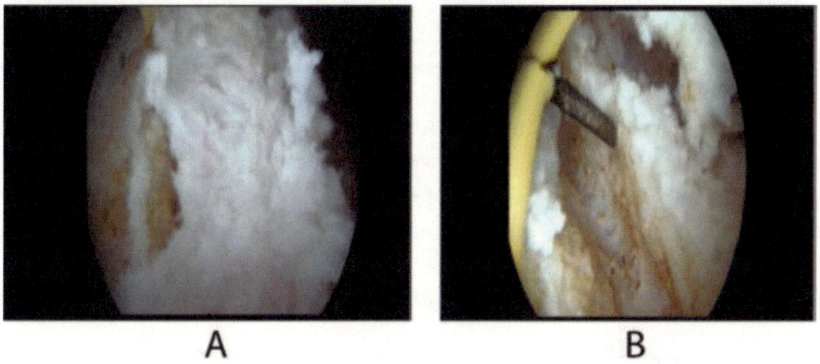


**Figure 9.** Hysteroscopic adhesiolysis: (A) resectoscopicadhesiolysis (hook electrode) and (B) scissors adhesiolysis.

## 2.14. ART for advanced pelvic adhesions

The endoscopist should be honest and document the post-CS findings meticulously. In extensive cases, he should counsel the couple for IVF/ICSI to save their time and money.

## 2.15. Topics related to CS that would affect future fertility

### *2.15.1. Isthmocele and infertility*

#### *2.15.1.1. Definition and incidence of isthmocele*

Isthmocele, endometrial reservoir, uterine niche or LSCS uterine scar dehiscence (CSD) are synonyms of the same disease which is discontinuation of the myometrium at the site of a previous CS. Simply, they describe a condition of deficiency of a part of lower segment CS scar as diagnosed in between pregnancies. This section will not cover uterine dehiscence during pregnancy and how to predict. Meta-analysis reports have shown the incidence of cesarean scar dehiscence to be around 1.9% [41]. The incidence of uterine niche irrespective of cause is around 0.6% worldwide [42]. On evaluation of 32 trials, cesarean scar defects are commonly found on ultrasound examination (24–88%) [43].

#### *2.15.1.2. What is the exact cause of isthmocele?*

Definitely it develops at the scar of previous CS. Thus, CS is the principal cause of this condition of incompletely healed scar. But why develops in some women, this is a matter of suggestions. The cause may be surgical fault in the form of bad surgical technique like closure of the hysterotomy incision using a single later technique, bad suturing material with marked inflammatory reaction, nontightness of continuous sutures, missing the endometrium during suturing, missing a part of the scar, very wide sutures or other possible defective surgical steps. Others suggested underlying anatomical defects in the uterus which would have been corrected prior to pregnancy like uterine septum or fibroid uterus may weaken the uterus and the resultant scar of the cesarean section [44]. Postoperative infection is an important contributing factor. Vervoort et al. [45] suggested that the possible factors that could play a role in niche development include a very low incision through cervical tissue, inadequate suturing technique during closure of the uterine scar, surgical interventions that increase adhesion formation or patient-related factors that impair wound healing or increase inflammation or adhesion formation.

#### *2.15.1.3. Predisposing factors for isthmocele formation*

Typical important causes would be previous lower segment cesarean section, classical cesarean section, previous uterine trauma, congenital anomaly, abnormal placenta implantation, and inappropriate oxytocin administration. Additional factors applicable to many patients would be nulliparity, diabetes, emergency surgery, infection, and incision placed too low in the uterine segment.

#### *2.15.1.4. Risk and probable factors for niche development*

Risk factors could be classified into four categories: those related to closure technique, to development of the lower uterine segment or location of the incision or to wound healing, and miscellaneous factors. Probable risk factors are single-layer myometrium closure, multiple CSs, and uterine retroflexion [46]. Others hypothesized some possible factors that could play a role in niche development including a very low incision through cervical tissue, inadequate suturing technique during closure of the uterine scar, surgical interventions that increase adhesion formation or patient-related factors that impair wound healing or increase inflammation or adhesion formation [45].

#### *2.15.2. Types of isthmocele*

Uterine dehiscence is of two types—complete and incomplete dehiscence. In incomplete uterine dehiscence, the myometrium is disrupted, but the serosa is intact. Full thickness tears of uterine wall result in complete uterine ruptures. These ruptures mostly occur at the level of previous cesarean section scars. Compared to complete uterine rupture, uterine dehiscence has much lower maternal and neonatal morbidity [46].

##### *2.15.2.1. Forms of isthmocele*

There is no universally agreed classification of isthmocele. It can be mild and severe. Severe is defined as the loss of >50% of myometrial mantle at the scar level [47]. A depth accounting for 80% or more of the muscle layer in the anterior wall of the uterus was referred to as "dehiscence." [48]

##### *2.15.2.2. Impact of isthmocele (niche) on woman's health*

Approximately 30% of women with a niche report spotting at 6–12 months after their CS. Other reported symptoms in women with a niche are dysmenorrhoea, chronic pelvic pain, and dyspareunia. Subfertility is an important sequence [49]. The association between a niche and gynecologic symptoms, obstetric complications, and potentially with subfertility highlights the importance of its prevention and proper management.

##### *2.15.2.3. How does isthmocele cause women's symptoms?*

The flow of menstrual blood through the cervix may be slowed by the presence of isthmocele, as the blood may accumulate in the niche because of the presence of fibrotic tissue, causing pelvic pain in the suprapubic area. Moreover, persistence of the menstrual blood after menstruation in the cervix may negatively influence the mucus quality and sperm quality, obstruct sperm transport through the cervical canal, interfere with embryo implantation, leading to secondary infertility [49].

##### *2.15.2.4. Clinical presentations of isthmocele*

The presentations are variable from silent to symptomatic. Main symptoms include dysmenorrhea, intermenstrual bleeding, irregular genital bleeding, chronic pelvic pain, dyspareunia, and secondary infertility [43]. Among the 293 patients diagnosed with CSD by transvaginal-sonography, the most common symptom was intermenstrual spotting (64%), followed by dysmenorrhea (53%), chronic pelvic pain (40%), and dyspareunia (18%) [50]. The most serious symptom is impending rupture uterus in late pregnancy. Isthmocele may present with post-partum hemorrhage, endomyometritis, and peritonitis (generalized/localized). Once peritonitis occurs as a result, sepsis may ensue risking the life of the patient [43]. Rare and unusual presentations have been reported in associations with wound infections, secondary PPH, concurrent postpartum uterine and abdominal wall dehiscence, site of implantation for ectopic pregnancy, etc. Infections with Streptococcus anginosus and Staphylococcus aureus have been reported also indicating the wide spectrum of infection possible in such a circumstance [43].

Scar tissue dehiscence, scar pregnancy, and abnormally adherent placenta are some of the obstetric complications associated with this defect [51].

*2.15.2.5. Isthmocele and infertility*

Is isthmocele a direct cause of infertility? The exact correlation is not yet settled in literature and requires more intensive studies of women with post-CS secondary infertility. Possible mechanism includes persistence of the menstrual blood after menstruation in the cervix which may negatively influence the mucus quality and sperm quality, obstruct sperm transport through the cervical canal, and interfere with embryo implantation [49]. As an initial proof of isthmocele-induced infertility, some nonrandomized studies reported high pregnancy rate after proper management of isthmocele. Seven out of 9 patients with secondary infertility became pregnant after hysteroscopic treatment (resection and roller-ball coagulation) [52].

*2.15.2.6. Diagnostic aids of isthmocele*

Transvaginal ultrasonography (TVS) with or without saline infusion hysterography (SIS) is usually quite sufficient for the diagnosis. TVS (**Figure 10**) shows an anechoic fluid-filled irregular defect seen at the anterior uterine isthmus, in relation to the site of a CS scar [53].

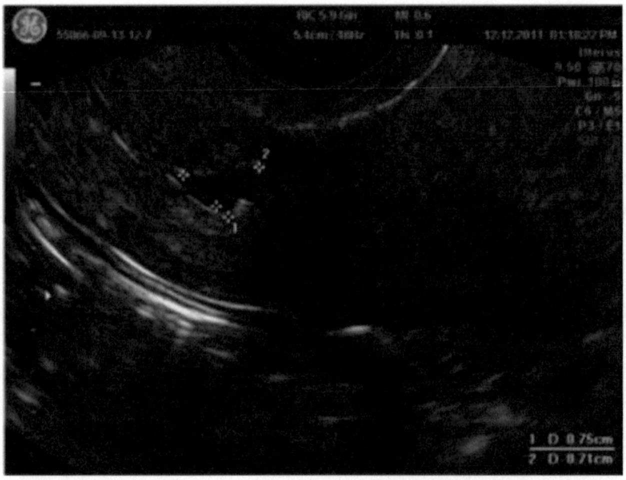

**Figure 10.** 2D TVS view of isthmocele at the scar site.

SIS can easily diagnose isthmocele by observing fluid accumulation in a reservoir at the site of previous CS scar. In selected cases, MRI may be ordered to complete the diagnosis particularly if the uterus is attracted upward by scars of previous CS(s), obese patients, posterior uterine wall defects after myomectomy, or if the size of the defect is not well defined. An important advantage of MRI is to detect the exact relationship between the defect and the urinary bladder prior to invasive endoscopic correction particularly in women with repeat CS.

### 2.15.2.7. *Treatment of isthmocele*

Basically, if there is no symptoms, no treatment but only follow-up before and during subsequent pregnancy for fear of scar dehiscence. Do not ignore the role of assurance, medical treatment, for example, BS antibiotic and symptomatic treatment, for example, diosmin and tranxamic acid for spotting treatments prior to rushing to surgical intervention. Treatment of uterine scar defects should be performed after eliminating other causes of postmenstrual bleeding or infertility [43]. Conservative management of infected isthmocele can be very successful and save the patient from invasive risky surgical procedures [54].

Treatment depends on the clinical presentation, parity, surgical risks, and the need for further children (**Figure 11**). If the patient is symptomatic and completed her family with expected extensive adhesions and high attraction of the uterus, laparotomy would be the most suitable approach with a consent of hysterectomy whenever severe isthmocele infection with friable defect is intraoperatively diagnosed. Some authors performed vaginal nonendoscopic excision of isthmocele with clinical improvement in 85.9% (55/64) [55]. Transvaginal repair was considered a minimal invasiveness procedure with good exposure and accurate resection [56]. Contradictally, these studies reported a prolonged operative time and postoperative stay (operation time was 67 ± 12 min, the mean blood loss was 53 ± 32 ml, and the mean length of hospital stay was 4.0 ± 1.1 days) which are against minimally invasive concept. Some surgeons rely on hysteroscopic confirmation and localization of isthmocele then proceed for vaginal nonendoscopic closure in two layers with good results [57].

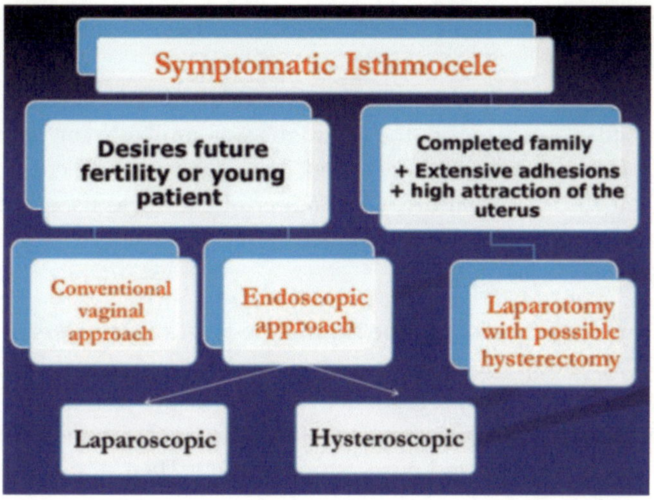


**Figure 11.** Management plan of symptomatizing isthmocele.

Endoscopic management is an attractive approach if fertility is concerned, patient is young, surgery is feasible, and probably, safe and endoscopist expertise is sufficient.

The question is to use laparoscopy or hysteroscopy for excision of this defect. Since studies are mainly case reports or small sample sized, the answer is not clear so far. Some studies stratified patients according to the uterine defect thickness. They considered women who desire future pregnancies and had a residual myometrial thickness of <3.5 mm or a defect that accounted for ≥50% of the anterior uterine wall, and laparoscopic surgical repair was performed with good postoperative anatomic outcomes. Women with residual myometrial thickness of ≥3.5 mm or a defect that accounted for <50% of the anterior uterine wall can be treated with hysteroscopic surgery to relief of symptoms [58]. However, others considered laparoscopic approach would increase uterine wall thickness when compared to hysteroscopic approach, and both surgical techniques seem to be effective for the resolution of gynecologic symptoms. Hysteroscopic treatment most likely corrects the scar defect but does not strengthen the uterine wall; thus, the potential risk of dehiscence or rupture in subsequent pregnancies does not seem to be improved. Because large uterine defects are known risk factors for scar dehiscence, laparoscopic repair of the defect to reinforce the myometrial endurance is warranted [59].

In a recent systematic review, hysteroscopic repair of a cesarean scar defect or isthmoplasty was associated with an improvement in uterine bleeding in 59–100% of cases and a pregnancy rate of 77.8–100%. An improvement in uterine bleeding after vaginal repair occurred in 89–93.5% of cases. Laparoscopic repair led to uterine bleeding improvement in 86% of cases and a pregnancy rate of 86%. Hysteroscopic isthmoplasty appears to be the most popular treatment [43].

Laparoscopic management has been described in many papers. It starts by careful dissection and freeing of the densely adherent bladder lower uterine segment. The defect is then localized with a sharp curette placed transcervically into the uterus. The curette pushes anteriorly to delineate the margins of the defect and puncture the ceiling of the isthmocele cavity. The fibrotic tissue that forms the ceiling and the lateral borders of the defect is excised using laparoscopic scissors. Lastly, reapproximation of the edges is done with continuous nonlocking 3-0 V-Loc sutures [51].

Others claim that robotic surgery would be more precise and accurate than conventional surgery [60]. As described in a case report, the technique was similar to conventional laparoscopy as the scar tissue around the defect is resected, and the freshened edges of the defect are closed using delayed absorbable suture. Chromopertubation was used to confirm the water tightness of the repair [60]. The same robotic technique was used to treat ectopic pregnancy implanted in an isthmocele [61].

Whether hysteroscopic resection of uterine isthmocele at least 3 mm versus no intervention is under evaluation in a multicentric study [62]. Hysteroscopic treatment of isthmocele is usually performed utilizing the resectoscope. It starts by hysteroscopic resection of the edges and the bottom of the defect until the complete removal of the fibrotic scar tissue showing the muscular tissue below, using a cutting loop and pure cutting current. Then, aimed electrocoagulation of the bottom of the pouch with a roller-ball is done to avoid the in situ production of blood [52].

To recapitulate, isthmocele has a definite impact on women's health. Preventive measures include overcoming predisposing factors. Performing CS in a microsurgical way as described in detail in this chapter would avoid exposing many women to this debatable disease. To treat or not to treat isthmocle and by which approach requires more studies according to the clinical situation particularly in case of post-CS infertility.

*2.15.2.8. Impact of cesarean myomectomy (CM) on future fertility*

Despite not universally agreed, some obstetricians are courageous and perform myomectomy for even multiple fibroids during CS [63, 64]. Personally, since a long time, I practice the technique of cesarean myomectomy with safe and satisfactory results. Many advantages of CM include elimination of the need for another laparotomy and another hysterotomy (uterine incision) and minimize the postpartum complications of fibroid including hemorrhage, torsion, and infection. A pregnant uterus is not always an obstacle for concomitant CM. The procedure is always preceded by IV administration of 1 g of tranexamic acid half an hour preoperatively. Bilateral uterine artery ligation is always done in all cases before myomectomy. In many cases, the access to the myoma can be done via intramyometrial incision through the cesarean hysterotomy incision, that is, no additional incision is required. We usually make an incision with the cutting diathermy till reaching the myoma which can be easily extracted with a towel forceps with insignificant bleeding from the bed. An important issue is the physiologic changes of the uterus on postpartum involution. A separate myomectomy scar at CS would be smaller by at least its half-length on uterine involution. High vascularity of the gravid uterus would help rapid and complete healing without defective scar seen after conventional myomectomy [65]. Last postulated positive point is that lower adhesions formation after CM due to pregnancy peculiar characteristics (see the beginning of this chapter). Nevertheless, the majority of obstetricians are against CM for fear of excessive uncontrollable bleeding that may require blood transfusion. The question is how excessive bleeding occurs and both uterine arteries are already ligated prior to CM. Moreover, the use of electrosurgery can control any bleeding point or vessel in no time. Lastly, uterine tourniquet is an excellent back up if bleeding is remarkable. Since studies on this topic are scarce, so far no available data on the future fertility after CM as this requires a randomized study of different sizes, sites, and number of fibroids. To be safer and fertility-oriented, without evidence, the obstetrician should follow adhesions preventive measures and fix an adhesion-preventive sheet over any separate myomectomy scar after CM.

*2.15.3. Placenta accrete and future fertility*

Placenta accreta is a potentially life-threatening obstetric condition that requires a multidisciplinary approach to management. The incidence of placenta accreta has increased and seems to parallel the increasing CD rate. Women at greatest risk of placenta accreta are those who have myometrial damage caused by a previous CD with either an anterior or posterior placenta previa overlying the uterine scar [66].

In many cases, the future fertility of those women will be compromised due to the aggressive manoeuvres to control bleeding, possibility of incomplete removal of the placenta, and the high liability to cesarean hysterectomy. Surgical treatment of placenta previa may compromise future fertility. One study reported secondary amenorrhea due to IUAs in 8 out of 96 women treated for placenta previa (8.3%) [67].

### *2.15.4. Post-CS scar secondary endometriosis*

Endometriosis can be primary or secondary which develops after surgery. In a very big study on postpartum endometriosis, 709,090 women were included [68]. New cases of endometriosis were noted in 3110 (0.4%). Women who had a CS were 80% more likely than women who had a vaginal delivery to receive an in-hospital diagnosis of endometriosis after delivery of their first child (hazard ratio, 1.8; 95% confidence interval, 1.7–1.9). The risk of endometriosis does not increase with the number of cesarean deliveries. The risk of endometriosis increased over time, with 1 additional case of endometriosis occurring for every 325 women who underwent a CS in a 10-year period. However, there was no dose-response effect, meaning that endometriosis was no more likely to develop in women who had 2 or more cesarean deliveries than in women who had just 1 cesarean delivery. The overall risk of endometriosis developing after CS remains very low. Other more common maternal risks related to CS include infection, blood loss requiring transfusion, and deep vein thrombosis or pulmonary embolism. The long-term risks of CS include uterine rupture of the incision site and problems with the position or type of placental growth in future pregnancies. Generally, a triad consisting of underlying mass at the incision, cyclic menstrual scar pain, and history of previous gynecological or obstetric surgery leads to the preoperative diagnosis [69].

The most common symptom of endometriosis after CS is the formation of a painful mass or lump of variable sizes in the surgical scar. Characteristically, both pain and size increase before and during menstruation due to bleeding inside the mass. Continuously, this mass irritates the adjacent tissues causing more pain and inflammation. The mass is discolored and even bleeds. Bleeding can be very confusing after giving CS. Sometimes, the mass is painless. Diagnosis is mainly clinically by palpation of a tender cystic mass or a firm mass if fibrosed at CS scar site with restricted mobility. High-resolution ultrasonography can detect the nature of the mass in many cases. Rarely, CT or MRI is ordered to confirm the diagnosis and to exclude other parietal masses. Nevertheless, the most reliable method to diagnose secondary endometriosis is tissue biopsy. Medications don't usually work for surgical scar endometriosis. Surgery is the first-line treatment of this mass, and postoperative medication might reduce recurrence [70]. After surgery, the chances that endometriosis will come back are small. Women who choose surgery have a very low recurrence rate.

## 2.16. Keynote points

- Despite pass smoothly in most cases, CS may compromise future fertility of women.
- Proper counseling for CS should stress on impact of CS on future fertility and the possibility of adhesion formation with subsequent endoscopic intervention or even assisted reproduction.
- Women awareness about other long-term complications of CS-like isthmocele, placenta previa, CS scar endometriosis, and possible cesarean hysterectomy should be highlighted.

- Doctor awareness about the importance of microsurgical steps of CS would minimize or even eliminate some long-term sequele of CS that would compromise women's health including future fertility.
- Additional procedures during CS require peculiar adhesion prevention precautions.

## Author details

Atef Darwish

Address all correspondence to: atef_darwish@yahoo.com

Woman's Health University Hospital, Assiut, Egypt

## References

[1] The American College of Obstetricians and Gynecologists (the College), the Society for Maternal-Fetal Medicine, Caughey AB, Cahill AG, Guise JM, Rouse DJ, MSPH. Obstetric Care Consensus. No 1, March 2014 (reaffirmed 2016).

[2] Boyle A, Reddy UM. Epidemiology of cesarean delivery: the scope of the problem. Semin Perinatol. 2012 Oct;36(5):308–14.

[3] WHO, HRP. WHO statement on caesarean section rates. Executive summary. April 2015, WHO/RHR/15.02, 1–8.

[4] Betrán A, Ye J, Moller A, Jun Zhang J, Gülmezoglu M, Torloni MR. The increasing trend in caesarean section rates: global, regional and national estimates: 1990–2014. PLoS One. 2016;11(2):e0148343.

[5] Awonuga AO, Fletcher NM, Saed GM, Diamond MP. Postoperative adhesion development following cesarean and open intra-abdominal gynecological operations: a review. Reprod Sci. 2011 Dec;18(12):1166–85.

[6] Berghella V. Cesarean delivery: technique. up to date 2016.

[7] Brill AI, Nezhat F, Nezhat CH, Nezhat C. The incidence of adhesions after prior laparotomy: a laparoscopic appraisal. Obstet Gynecol. 1995;85(2):269–72.

[8] Ashrafinia M, Vazirichimeh Z, Dastjerdi MV, Moiini A. Adhesion formation in patients with previous laparotomies. J Am Assoc Gynecol Laparosc. 1996;3(4 suppl):S2.

[9] Clark EA, Silver RM. Long-term maternal morbidity associated with repeat cesarean delivery. Am J Obstet Gynecol. 2011;205(6 Suppl):S2–10.

[10] Gurol-Urganci I, Bou-Antoun S, Lim CP, Cromwell DA, Mahmood TA, Templeton A, van der Meulen JH. Impact of caesarean section on subsequent fertility: a systematic review and meta-analysis. Hum Reprod. 2013;28(7):1943–52.

[11] Alpay et al. Semin Reprod Med. 2008;26:289–297, 313–221.

[12] Juntunen K, Makarainen L, Kirkinen P. Outcome after a high number (4–10) of repeated caesarean sections. BJOG. 2004;111(6):561–563

[13] Kelly J Morales, Michael C Gordon, Gordon Wright Bates. Postcesarean delivery adhesions associated with delayed delivery of infant. Am J Obstetrics Gynecol. 2007;196(5):461.e1–6.

[14] Ben-Nagi J, Walker A, Jurkovic D, Yazbek J, Aplin JD. Effect of cesarean delivery on the endometrium. Int J Gynaecol Obstet. 2009;106(1):30–4.

[15] Gonzalez-Quintero VH, Cruz-Pachano FE. Preventing adhesions in obstetric and gynecologic surgical procedures. Rev Obstet Gynecol. 2009;2(1):38–45

[16] Memon S, Qazi RA, Bibi S, Parveen N. Effect of preoperative vaginal cleaning with an antiseptic solution to reduce post cesarean infectious morbidity. J Pak Med Assoc. 2011;61(12):1179–83.

[17] Salama FA, Yehia AH, Wahba KA, Abdelmoniem RM. Efficacy and safety of chlorhexidine versus povidone-iodine skin antisepsis in reducing surgical site infection in cesarean sections: a randomized, controlled clinical trial. Evid Based Women's Health J. 2016;6(1):32–36.

[18] Smaill FM, Grivell RM. Routine antibiotics at cesarean section to reduce infection. Cochrane Rep. 2014.

[19] Dahlke JD, Mendez-Figueroa H, Rouse DJ, et al. Evidence-based surgery for cesarean delivery: an updated systematic review. Am J Obstet Gynecol. 2013;209:294.

[20] Mathai M, Hofmeyr GJ. Abdominal surgical incisions for caesarean section. Cochrane Database Syst Rev. 2007; CD004453.

[21] Hofmeyr JG, Novikova N, Mathai M, Shah A. Techniques for cesarean section. Am J Obstet Gynecol. 2009;201:431.

[22] Magann EF, Chauhan SP, Bufkin L, et al. Intra-operative haemorrhage by blunt versus sharp expansion of the uterine incision at caesarean delivery: a randomised clinical trial. BJOG. 2002;109:448.

[23] Hohlagschwandtner M, Ruecklinger E, Husslein P, Joura EA. Is the formation of a bladder flap at cesarean necessary? A randomized trial. Obstet Gynecol. 2001;98:1089.

[24] Tuuli MG, Odibo AO, Fogertey P, et al. Utility of the bladder flap at cesarean delivery: a randomized controlled trial. Obstet Gynecol. 2012;119:815.

[25] Zaphiratos V, George RB, Boyd JC, Habib AS. Uterine exteriorization compared with in situ repair for Cesarean delivery: a systematic review and meta-analysis. Can J Anaesth. 2015;62:1209.

[26] Yazicioglu F, Gökdogan A, Kelekci S, et al. Incomplete healing of the uterine incision after caesarean section: Is it preventable? Eur J Obstet Gynecol Reprod Biol. 2006;124:32.

[27] Roberge S, Demers S, Berghella V, et al. Impact of single- vs double-layer closure on adverse outcomes and uterine scar defect: a systematic review and metaanalysis. Am J Obstet Gynecol 2014;211:453.

[28] Yasmin S, Sadaf J, Fatima N. Impact of methods for uterine incision closure on repeat caesarean section scar of lower uterine segment. J Coll Physicians Surg Pak. 2011;21: 522.

[29] Ceci O, Cantatore C, Scioscia M, et al. Ultrasonographic and hysteroscopic outcomes of uterine scar healing after cesarean section: comparison of two types of single-layer suture. J Obstet Gynaecol Res. 2012;38:1302.

[30] Roberge S, Chaillet N, Boutin A, et al. Single- versus double-layer closure of the hysterotomy incision during cesarean delivery and risk of uterine rupture. Int J Gynaecol Obstet. 2011;115:5.

[31] Kapustian V, Anteby EY, Gdalevich M, et al. Effect of closure versus nonclosure of peritoneum at cesarean section on adhesions: a prospective randomized study. Am J Obstet Gynecol. 2012;206:56.e1.

[32] Cheong YC, Premkumar G, Metwally M, et al. To close or not to close? A systematic review and a meta-analysis of peritoneal non-closure and adhesion formation after caesarean section. Eur J Obstet Gynecol Reprod Biol. 2009;147:3.

[33] Shi Z, Ma L, Yang Y, et al. Adhesion formation after previous caesarean section-a meta-analysis and systematic review. BJOG. 2011;118:410.

[34] Gates S, Anderson ER. Wound drainage for caesarean section. Cochrane Database Syst Rev. 2013;12:CD004549.

[35] CAESAR study collaborative group. Caesarean section surgical techniques: a randomised factorial trial (CAESAR). BJOG. 2010;117:1366.

[36] Ramsey PS, White AM, Guinn DA, et al. Subcutaneous tissue reapproximation, alone or in combination with drain, in obese women undergoing cesarean delivery. Obstet Gynecol. 2005;105:967.

[37] De Wilde RL, Brölmann H, Robert Koninckx P, Lundorff P, Lower AM, Wattiez A, Mara M, Wallwiener M. Prevention of adhesions in gynaecological surgery: the 2012 European field guideline. Gynecol Surg. 2012 Nov;9(4):365–368.

[38] Bateman BG, Nunley WC, Kitchin JV III. Surgical management of distal tubal obstruction- Are we making progress? Fertil Steril. 1987;48:523–542.

[39] DeWilde RL, Trew G. Postoperative abdominal adhesions and their prevention in gynaecological surgery. Expert consensus position. Part 2—steps to reduce adhesions. Gynecol Surg. 2007;4:243–253.

[40] Committee on Obstetric Practice. Cesarean Delivery on Maternal Request 2013. No 559.

[41] Tahara M, Shimizu T, Shimoura H. Preliminary report of treatment with oral contraceptive pills for intermenstrual vaginal bleeding secondary to a cesarean section scar. Fertil Steril. 2006;86(2):477–9.

[42] Diaz SD, Jones JE, Seryakov M, Mann WJ. Uterine rupture and dehiscence: ten-year review and case control study. South Med J. 2002;95:431–5.

[43] Tulandi T, Cohen A. Emerging manifestations of cesarean scar defect in reproductive-aged women. J Minim Invasive Gynecol. 2016 Sep–Oct;23(6):893–902.

[44] Bharatam KK. Cesarean section uterine scar dehiscence—a review. Uterus Ovary 2015;2:e751.

[45] Vervoort AJ, Uittenbogaard LB, Hehenkamp WJ, Brölmann HA, Mol BW, Huirne JA. Why do niches develop in Caesarean uterine scars? Hypotheses on the aetiology of niche development. Hum Reprod. 2015;30(12):2695–702.

[46] Bij de Vaate AJ, van der Voet LF, Naji O, Witmer M, Veersema S, Brölmann HA, Bourne T, Huirne JA. Prevalence, potential risk factors for development and symptoms related to the presence of uterine niches following Cesarean section: systematic review. Ultrasound Obstet Gynecol. 2014;43(4):372–82.

[47] Ofili-Yebovi D, Ben Nagi J, Sawyer E, et al. Deficient low-segment cesarean section scars: prevalence and risk factors. Ultrasound Obstet Gynecol 2008;31:72–77.

[48] Osser OV, Jokubkiene L, Valentin L. Cesarean section scar defects: agreement between transvaginalsonographic findings with and without saline contrast enhancement. Ultrasound Obstet Gynecol. 2010;35:75–83.

[49] Florio P, Filippeschi M, Moncini I, Gubbini G. Hysteroscopic treatment of the cesarean-induced isthmocele in restoring infertility. Curr Opin Obstet Gynecol. 2012;24(3): 180–6.

[50] Wagner MS, Bédard MJ. Postpartum uterine wound dehiscence: a case report. J Obstet Gynaecol Can. 2006;28:713–715.

[51] Urman B, Arslan T, Aksu S, Taskiran C. Laparoscopic repair of cesarean scar defect "isthmocele". J Minim Invasive Gynecol. 2016;23(6):857–8.

[52] Gubbini G, Casadio P, Marra E. Resectoscopic correction of the "isthmocele" in women with postmenstrual abnormal uterine bleeding and secondary infertility. J Minim Invasive Gynecol. 2008;15(2):172–5.

[53] Savelli L, Scifo M, Gubbini G. P23.04: Sonographic features of Caesarean-induced isthmocele before and after resectoscopic correction in symptomatic non-pregnant women. Ultrasound Obstet Gynecol. 2016;48(S1):241–242.

[54] Boukrid M, Dubuisson J. Conservative Management of a Scar Abscess formed in a Cesarean-induced Isthmocele. Front Surg. 2016;3:7.

[55] Chen Y, Chang Y, Yao S. Transvaginal management of cesarean scar section diverticulum: a novel surgical treatment. Med Sci Monit. 2014;20:1395–9.

[56] Yao M, Chen H, Tao J, Li Y, Sun M, Zhu J, Chen P, Wang X. Clinical research of transvaginal repair of cesarean scar diverticulum. Zhonghua Fu Chan KeZaZhi. 2015;50(7):500–4.

[57] Luo L, Niu G, Wang Q, Xie HZ, Yao SZ.Vaginal repair of cesarean section scar diverticula. J Minim Invasive Gynecol. 2012;19(4):454–8.

[58] Li C, Guo Y, Liu Y, Cheng J, Zhang W. Hysteroscopic and laparoscopic management of uterine defects on previous cesarean delivery scars. J Perinat Med. 2014;42(3):363–70.

[59] Api M, Boza A, Gorgen H, Api O. Should cesarean scar defect be treated laparoscopically? A case report and review of the literature. J Minim Invasive Gynecol. 2015;22(7): 1145–52.

[60] Mahmoud MS, Nezhat FR. Robotic-assisted laparoscopic repair of a cesarean section scar defect. J Minim Invasive Gynecol. 2015;22(7):1135–6.

[61] Schmitt A, Crochet P, Agostini A. Robotic-assisted laparoscopic treatment of residual ectopic pregnancy in a previous cesarean section scar: a case report. J Minim Invasive Gynecol. 2016. pii: S1553–4650(16)31006–8.

[62] Vervoort A, Van der Voet L, WitmerM, Thurkow A, Radder C, van Kesteren, Quartero H, Kuchenbecker W, Bongers M et al. The HysNiche trial: hysteroscopic resection of uterine caesarean scar defect (niche) in patients with abnormal bleeding, a randomised controlled trial BMC Women's Health. 2015;15:103.

[63] Roman AS, Tabsh KM. Myomectomy at time of cesarean delivery: a retrospective cohort study. BMC Pregnancy Childbirth. 2004;4:14.

[64] Bhatla N, Dash B, Kriplani A, Agarwal N. Myomectomy during pregnancy: a feasible option. J Obstet Gynaecol Res. 2009;35(1):173–175.

[65] Darwish AM, Nasr AM, El-Nashar DA. Evaluation of postmyomectomy uterine scars. J Clin Ultrasound. 2005;26;33(4):181–186.

[66] ACOG Committee opinion: Placenta Accreta Number 529, July 2012. Reaffirmed 2015.

[67] Sentilhes L, Kayem G, Ambroselli C, Provansal M, Fernandez H, Perrotin F, Winer N, Pierre F, Benachi A, Dreyfus M, Bauville E, Mahieu-Caputo D, Marpeau L, Descamps P, Bretelle F, Goffinet F. Fertility and pregnancy outcomes following conservative treatment for placenta accreta. Hum Reprod. 2010;25(11):2803–10.

[68] Andolf E, Thorsell M, Kallen K. Caesarean section and risk for endometriosis: a prospective cohort study of Swedish registries. BJOG. 2013. doi:10.1111/1471-0528.12236.

[69] Miccini M, Gregori M, Ferraro D, Ciardi A, Cassibba S, Biacchi D. Abdominal scar endometriosis: case report. Clin Exp Obstet Gynecol. 2016;43(3):431–3.

[70] Zhang J, Liu X. Clinicopathological features of endometriosis in abdominal wall—clinical analysis of 151 cases. Clin Exp Obstet Gynecol. 2016;43(3):379–83.

Section 2

# Fertility-oriented Hysteroscopic Surgery

Chapter 2

# Hysteroscopic Surgery for Submucosal Fibroids

Rashi Kalra and Roger J Hart

Additional information is available at the end of the chapter

http://dx.doi.org/10.5772/64861

**Abstract**

This chapter presents a contemporary summary of the evidence of the clinical impact of submucosal fibroids and discusses the methods used to investigate and surgically manage this common gynaecological condition.

**Keywords:** fibroid, submucosal fibroid, leiomyoma, female infertility, abnormal uterine bleeding, surgery, hysteroscopy, resectoscope, hysteroscopic surgery, menorrhagia, recurrent miscarriage

## 1. Introduction

Submucosal leiomyomas or fibroids are estimated to be the cause of 5–10% of cases of abnormal uterine bleeding, pain, subfertility and infertility [1].

This chapter focuses on the diagnostic methods to determine the type of submucosal leiomyomas present, their impact on uterine bleeding and infertility, and the methods used to resect these leiomyomas.

## 2. Classification of fibroids

It is important to classify fibroids according to the degree of endometrial cavity distortion when considering therapeutic options such as a surgical approach. The degree of intramural extension has implications for operative difficulty and risk. The most widely used system classifies submucous leiomyomas into three subtypes according to the proportion of the lesion's diameter that is within the myometrium as determined by saline infusion sonography (SIS) or hysteroscopy. Type 0 leiomyomas are completely intracavitary, type 1 leiomyomas are less than 50% intramural and type 2 leiomyomas more than 50% intramural [2, 3].

This classification has been shown to be predictive of the likelihood of complete surgical resection, which is the most predictive indicator of surgical success. Uterine size and the number of leiomyomas also have been shown to be independent prognostic variables for recurrence [2, 4].

A newer and more detailed classification system has been devised and advocated by the International Federation of Gynecology and Obstetrics (FIGO). This system allows for categorization of the relationship of the leiomyoma outer boundary with the uterine serosa, a relationship that is important when evaluating women suitable for resectoscopic surgery. Thus, a type 2 leiomyoma that reaches the serosa is considered to be a type 2–5 lesion and therefore not a candidate for resectoscopic surgery (see **Figure 1**).

**Leiomyoma subclassification system**

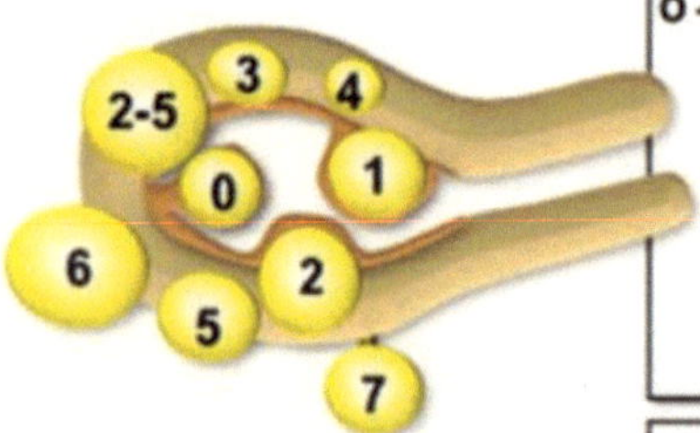


| | | |
|---|---|---|
| SM - Submucosal | 0 | Pedunculated intracavitary |
| | 1 | <50% intramural |
| | 2 | ≥50% intramural |
| O - Other | 3 | Contacts endometrium; 100% intramural |
| | 4 | Intramural |
| | 5 | Subserosal ≥50% intramural |
| | 6 | Subserosal <50% intramural |
| | 7 | Subserosal pedunculated |
| | 8 | Other (specify e.g. cervical, parasitic) |
| Hybrid leiomyomas (impact both endometrium and serosa) | Two numbers are listed separated by a hyphen. By convention, the first refers to the relationship with the endometrium while the second refers to the relationship to the serosa. One example is below | |
| | 2-5 | Submucosal and subserosal, each with less than half the diameter in the endometrial and peritoneal cavities, respectively. |

**Figure 1.** FIGO classification of submucous leiomyomas. Reproduced with permission granted by Elsevier.

## 2.1. Diagnostic methods for classifications of fibroids

The methods to confirm the presence of a submucous fibroid include ultrasonography (typically transvaginal ultrasonography, TVUS), saline infusion sonography (SIS), diagnostic hysteroscopy, hysterosalpingography and magnetic resonance imaging (MRI). The diagnosis

http://dx.doi.org/10.5772/64861

of submucous fibroids is generally achieved with one or a combination of hysteroscopy and radiological techniques. The aims are to distinguish leiomyomas from adenomyosis, confirmation of submucous location, as well the number, size, location and extent of myometrial penetration of each identified submucous myoma. The relationship of the submucous myoma to the uterine serosa is of particular importance as transcervical resection is not appropriate when the leiomyoma is very close to or in contact with the serosal layer of the uterus, due to an increased risk of uterine perforation and visceral injury with significant associated morbidity.

A surgeon can get the best appreciation for the location and relationship of submucosal fibroids to the uterine serosa by reviewing the radiological images themselves prior to the planned operation. This well help them decide the best approach to resecting the fibroids. The quality of the images obtained therefore plays a significant role. These imaging modalities will be discussed in detail below [5].

#### *2.1.1. Transvaginal ultrasonography (TVUS)*

TVUS has a sensitivity of 0.8 and a specificity of 0.7 for diagnosing submucous fibroids, and is generally thought to have limited use for exclusion of submucous fibroids and polyps (negative likelihood ratio 0.29) [6]. However, a prospective study suggested that when TVUS has been used as a first-step investigation, diagnostic hysteroscopy can be avoided in 40% of cases. This would suggest that it is a viable non-invasive initial investigation [6]. Unfortunately, TVUS is very operator dependent, a factor that must be considered when evaluating its reliability.

#### *2.1.2. Saline infusion sonography (SIS)*

Hysterosonography or saline infusion sonography (SIS) is a non-invasive imaging technique performed at the time of transvaginal ultrasound. Saline is introduced into the uterine cavity at the time of ultrasound and distends the uterine cavity to give better visualization of the endometrium and any intrauterine tumours or polyps [7].

The procedure is best performed when the endometrium is thin and the patient is not pregnant, therefore the first ten days of a menstrual cycle. The cervix is identified by speculum examination and a fine catheter inserted into the cervical os with a saline containing syringe at the end of the catheter. A transvaginal ultrasound is then performed at the same time as the injection of the saline. The procedure takes no more than 10–15 minutes. The benefit of saline infusion sonography is that the intramural component of a submucous fibroid is then better visualized by the ultrasound (see **Figure 2**) [5]. There is high-quality evidence from a Cochrane systematic review that demonstrates SIS and hysteroscopy to be equivalent for the diagnosis of submucous leiomyomas, with both superior to TVUS [8]. The main drawbacks of this technique are the risk of infection (1%) and the discomfort associated with injection of sterile saline into the uterus.

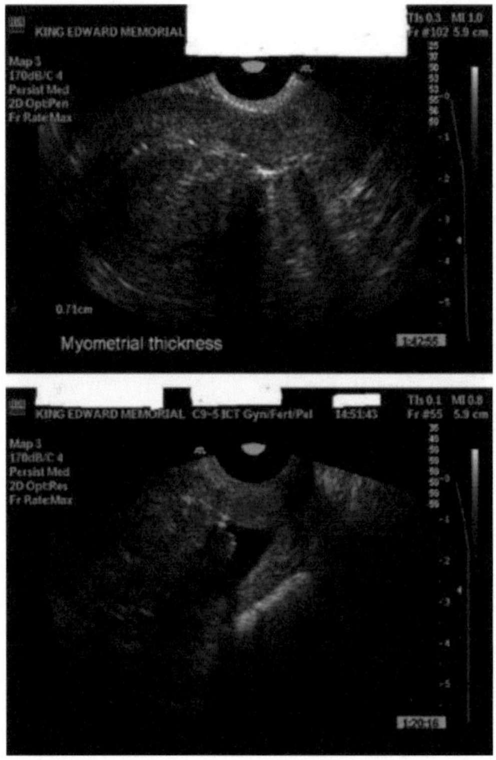


**Figure 2.** Ultrasound before and after instillation of saline as a contrast medium.

### *2.1.3. Diagnostic hysteroscopy*

Hysteroscopy involves inserting a telescope (usually 2.7–4 mm) into the endometrial cavity. The procedure may be performed in an outpatient setting without anaesthetic, even in nulliparous women and is highly successful, although some women (approximately 25%) will require local anaesthesia and some women may prefer general anaesthesia. If the patient requires a local anaesthetic, it can be administered by a paracervical block using 5 mL of 1% lignocaine. This can be injected at the level where a tenaculum is applied to the cervix and also at the 3 o′ clock and 9 o′ clock positions deep enough to the level of the internal cervical os. Other options are topical local anaesthetic gel, spray or cream [9, 10].

As for any procedure on the uterus it is essential to exclude the possibility of pregnancy and active infection. The administration of a non-steroidal anti-inflammatory prior to the procedure has been demonstrated to reduce the patient's posthysteroscopy discomfort [11].

Two methods of uterine distension are used—carbon dioxide and normal saline instillation. A randomized controlled trial (RCT) of carbon dioxide versus normal saline instillation during hysteroscopy found that normal saline provided comparable visualization to carbon dioxide with reduced procedure time and patient discomfort [12]. The distending pressure normally used is 80–100 mmHg.

Diagnostic hysteroscopy can be used to assess and document uterine abnormalities which should then be recorded by digital images. These can be used to plan an operative procedure and also facilitate the patient's understanding of their pathology (see **Figure 3**). The procedure should be performed quickly to avoid patient discomfort and manipulation of the cervix when rotating the hysteroscope should be avoided.

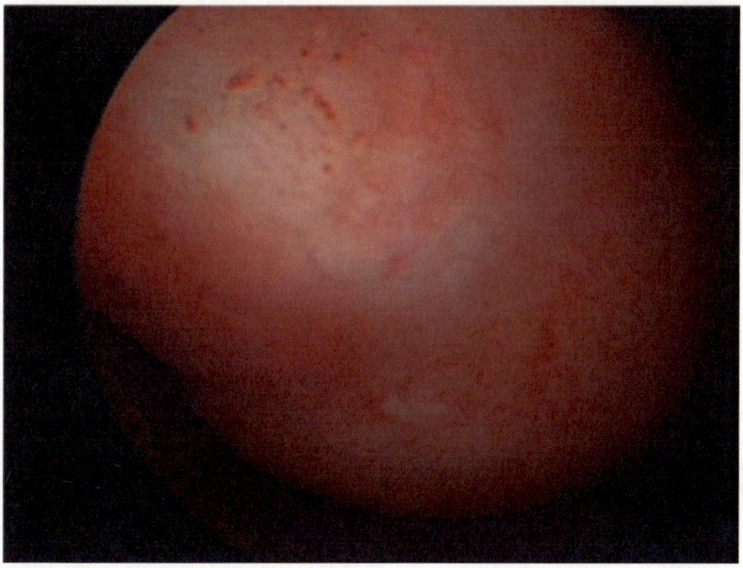

**Figure 3.** Hysteroscopic image of fibroid prior to resection.

### *2.1.4. Magnetic resonance imaging (MRI)*

Magnetic resonance imaging (MRI) is a costly imaging technique which is not available in all units. However, the use of T2-weighted images allows accurate localisation of the demarcation between the endometrium and myometrium. MRI is the most accurate modality in assessing the adnexae and the uterus because it provides information on the size, location, number and perfusion of leiomyomas as well as the presence of other uterine pathology including adenomyosis or endometriosis [13].

A double-blinded study demonstrated that although TVUS and MRI are roughly equivalent in diagnosing the presence of leiomyomas, the determination of other features such as location and proportion of the tumour in the endometrial cavity, is best accomplished with MRI. It was shown to be the most reliable method of evaluation when compared with vaginal ultrasound, hysterosonography and hysteroscopy, with 100% sensitivity and 91% specificity (gold standard was pathological examination) [14].

MRI was superior to the TVUS and SIS in evaluating the relationship of submucous leiomyomas to the myometrium [15]. MRI is becoming more available for the assessment of submucosal fibroids; however, the costs involved and its availability limit its use.

## 3. Indications for surgery

If a submucosal fibroid is confirmed with selected diagnostic modalities, the decision to operate should be individualized based on the patient and their symptoms. It is believed that one in three women with fibroids experience abnormal uterine bleeding (AUB) and that the presence of a submucosal fibroid increases the chance of this. The two most common indications for surgery are described below [16, 17].

### 3.1. Menorrhagia

There is little evidence implicating the role of FIGO staged submucous leiomyomas as the cause of haemorrhage requiring urgent intervention [18]. However, there is evidence to suggest that submucous leiomyomas can cause chronic abnormal uterine bleeding and heavy menstrual bleeding (HMB).

A systematic review of 11 studies demonstrated the prevalence of submucous myomas in women with AUB was 23.4%. Submucous myomas were found in 23.4% of premenopausal women (six studies) and 4.5% of postmenopausal women with AUB (one study). Although these studies fell short of proving that submucous myomas cause AUB they suggest that there may be a relationship. The incidence of submucous fibroids in 323 consecutive asymptomatic women undergoing sterilization was reported at 1.8%, whereas in a series of women with abnormal uterine bleeding, submucous fibroids were reported more frequently (6–34%) [19].

Broadbent and Magos [20], measured menstrual blood loss before and after hysteroscopic surgery of submucosal fibroids and showed that surgery improved both dysmenorrhea and heavy bleeding. They demonstrated that after surgery there was a significant reduction in the duration, blood loss and pain score associated with menstruation.

There are various theories for the pathophysiology of how submucous fibroids contribute to abnormal uterine bleeding and menorrhagia. It is thought that the mechanisms involved in haemostasis and prostaglandin production in the endometrium can be disturbed by the presence of fibroids. Another hypothesis is that it can be due to increased endometrial surface area of the endometrium. Both submucous and intramural fibroids have the potential to cause this [21].

### 3.2. Infertility

Women undergoing IVF treatment in the presence of a submucosal fibroid have lower clinical pregnancy rates than those without fibroids (10% vs. 30%) as seen in a retrospective comparative study of over 400 assisted reproductive treatment cycles. This may suggest an association between submucosal fibroids and subfertility. One major drawback was that in this study there were only nine patients in the submucosal fibroid group. Similar results were recorded in a study by Farhi et al. [22, 23]. There have been no appropriately designed studies to demonstrate a direct causal relationship between the presence of fibroids and infertility.

Many hypotheses have been generated to explain how fibroids might cause infertility. Perfusion studies have shown that blood flow to uterine fibroids is less than that to the adjacent myometrium. Blood flow to the uterine arteries is also different in a fibroid uterus than a non-fibroid uterus [24]. This and the fact that there may be endometrial inflammation and an altered local hormonal environment may affect embryo implantation. Myomas also seem to alter uterine contractility possibly interfering with sperm and ovum interaction or embryo migration [25]. This may especially be true in a uterus with multiple large fibroids with cavity distortion.

Six systematic reviews or meta-analyses published between 2001 and 2010 assessed whether fibroids have an impact on fertility. On the whole, it appears that women with fibroids have decreased fertility. The presence of fibroids, regardless of location, significantly decreases both implantation and clinical pregnancy rates (RR 0.821; 95% CI 0.722–0.932, $P = 0.002$ and RR 0.849; 95% CI 0.734–0.982, $P < 0.03$, respectively). The impact of fibroid number and size on fertility has not been clearly elucidated. Reproductive success does, however, seem to be related to fibroid location [26, 27].

All systematic reviews and meta-analyses agree that subserosal fibroids do not have an impact on fertility. Submucosal fibroids (fibroids with endometrial impingement), however, have been shown uniformly to have a negative impact on rates of implantation, clinical pregnancy rate, miscarriage and live birth/ongoing pregnancy, although available studies are few and small [24, 27].

In conclusion, submucosal fibroids are associated with reduced fertility and an increased miscarriage rate. Hysteroscopic myomectomy for submucosal fibroids is likely to improve fertility outcomes; however, the quality of available studies is poor and further research is required. The relative effect of multiple or different sized fibroids on fertility outcomes are also uncertain [28].

## 4. Surgical management of submucosal fibroids

Surgical resection remains the mainstay for women with symptomatic submucosal fibroids. Medical therapy with gonadotrophin-releasing hormone analogues (GnRHa) appears useful in the short term but side effects limit their long-term use [5]. Medical management of fibroids delays efforts to conceive and is not recommended for the management of infertility associated with fibroids. However, short-term GnRH analog use in infertile women with fibroids can be useful for preoperative correction of anaemia or short-term reduction in fibroid volume [28].

Newer, novel therapies including aromatase inhibitors, mifepristone, selective estrogen receptor modulators and selective progesterone receptor modulators have shown promise in symptom improvement and fibroid regression without the hypoestrogenic symptoms associated with GnRH analogues however they are currently only used in the setting of approved clinical trials on the management of fibroids in women with infertility.

The same applies to other alternatives to surgery such as uterine artery embolization (UAE), magnetic resonance-guided focused ultrasound surgery (MRgFUS), myolysis and radiofrequency ablation (RFA) all of which are still being investigated in terms of their long-term impact on fertility [24, 28].

### 4.1. Transcervical resectoscopic myomectomy (TCRM)

Transcervical resectoscopic myomectomy (TCRM) was performed in 1976 with a modified urologic resectoscope [29]. Traditionally, this has been the most common method of hysteroscopic resection of fibroids, but various new modalities such as vapourisation, morcellation and dissection are now being used in the surgical management of fibroids [3].

Hysteroscopic myomectomy is the least invasive surgical approach for fibroid removal. It is most effective for patients with submucosal fibroids completely within the uterine cavity (type 0) or with at least 50% of the fibroid volume within the uterine cavity (type 1). Fibroids with less than 50% of the fibroid volume in the cavity (type 2) are much more difficult to resect completely and are more often associated with the need for repeated procedures.

Submucous fibroids less than or equal to 5 cm diameter can be removed hysteroscopically however anything larger in diameter should be removed abdominally whether by laparoscopy or laparotomy (midline or pfannensteil) depending on surgeon's skill and preference. Type 2 fibroids tend to require a multi-staged procedure when compared to type 0 and 1 [4, 24].

#### *4.1.1. Patient selection*

Achievement of a high likelihood of surgical success requires good patient selection and relevant factors such as the number of submucous myomas, their location, size and type, and their relationship to the uterine serosa should be considered. When evaluating the suitability of patients for TCRM, it is important to consider the myoma type, the potential for incomplete excision and the patient's tolerance for more than one procedure if required. The indication for fibroid resection is also very important.

With resection of fibroids for abnormal bleeding, it is found that type 2 myomas could be eventually resected but required a larger number of repeat procedures than the more superficial types 0 and 1 myomas, which almost invariably are completed with a single operation [30, 31].

A recently published randomized controlled trial compared treatment of submucous myomas in 215 women with primary infertility. Fertility rates increased after TCRM for type 0 and type 1 myomas, but no significant difference was noted between the groups for type 2 myomas. However, a number of questions related to the effects of resection of myomas on fertility remain unanswered and highlight the need for careful patient selection in this population [32].

The same applies with regard to multiple pregnancy loss. Data from Pritts et al. suggest that in selected patients submucous myomectomy may reduce the rate of spontaneous abortion; however, more data are required to confirm this [27].

http://dx.doi.org/10.5772/64861

#### *4.1.2. Pre-operative preparation*

##### *4.1.2.1. Suppressive medical therapy before TCRM*

Commencing the patient on a gonadotrophin hormone-releasing (GnRH) analogue or selective progesterone receptor modulator (mifepristone or ulipristal acetate) [33] prior to the surgery allows the surgeon to operate when the endometrium is thin which can reduce operative time by allowing better visualization during the procedure. Theoretically, this also reduces intraoperative bleeding and fluid absorption. However, its main proven benefit is that it can reduce menstrual blood loss and correction of anaemia prior to surgery. This also aids with restoration of haemoglobin and iron stores for the woman. Whereas high-quality data exist demonstrating the efficacy of GnRH agonists in facilitating the treatment of anaemia before the procedure the data regarding the impact on other outcomes is more mixed, although the use of selective progesterone receptor blockers may show promise [34–36].

##### *4.1.2.2. Cervical preparation before TCRM*

Various methods are available for preoperative ripening of the cervix prior to hysteroscopic resection. The benefit of cervical ripening is to reduce the risk of cervical tears and uterine perforation that is associated with forceful dilatation. These risks are increased in postmenopausal women, for those without previous vaginal delivery and for women with previous surgery for cervical surgery or neoplasia. Options for ripening include laminaria tents, preoperative prostaglandins such as misoprostol and intraoperative intracervical injection of dilute vasopressin [3].

Probably the best available evidence is for use of prostaglandins. High-quality evidence from randomized controlled trials suggests that misoprostol, a synthetic prostaglandin $E_1$ analogue (200–400 mcg) taken orally or vaginally, 12–24 hours before surgery, facilitates cervical dilation and minimizes traumatic complications in premenopausal women [37]. The cervix is then usually dilated to accept a size 10 Hegar dilator.

##### *4.1.2.3. Prophylactic antibiotics and intra-operative preparation*

The risk of infection from hysteroscopic procedures is low, in the order of 0.5–1% with a risk of endometritis following resectoscopic myomectomy of 0.51% [38]. Most operators would however routinely administer prophylactic antibiotics to limit postoperative febrile morbidity, although there is no prospective data to support this practice.

##### *4.1.2.4. Anaesthesia*

Resection of a submucosal fibroid is usually performed after the administration of general anaesthetic, although it may be performed with spinal anaesthesia or with local anaesthetic; paracervical block and intrauterine injection of local anaesthetic in association with intravenous sedation [39].

Increasingly over the last decade, more operative hysteroscopic procedures have been performed in an office-based setting. Mcilwaine et al. showed in a study of 42 patients that the

Myosure lite device (uses electromechanical energy) can be successfully used to resect small fibroids in the outpatient setting with a high level of patient satisfaction with the use of local anaesthetic in a paracervical block [40].

### 4.2. Surgical technique

Patients are generally placed in lithotomy position: Trendelenburg positioning should be avoided. After an examination under anaesthesia, a bivalve speculum is placed in the vagina and the cervix identified. After placing a single tooth tenaculum on the anterior lip of the cervix (if the patient is conscious local anaesthetic spray can be applied prior to this), the cervix is dilated with Hegar dilators to size 10 sufficient to accommodate the 9 mm outer sheath of a standard resectoscope. The longer dilators with a gradually tapered tip are safer and minimize the risk of perforation [41].

The correct and safe use of instruments available will enable the surgeon to most effectively carry out hysteroscopic fibroid resection. In the past, smaller fibroids have been removed with conventional instruments such as grasping polyp forceps or scissors; however, there is now a growing trend towards performing the procedure with devices under direct vision [3]. They have the added benefit of early recognition of the complication of uterine perforation and reducing its associated morbidity.

#### *4.2.1. Hysteroscopic systems*

For optimum safety and effectiveness, the surgeon should have a detailed understanding of the design and assembly, and where necessary, troubleshooting strategies for the system in use.

The most commonly employed system for removal of submucous myomas is the urologic resectoscope, slightly modified for gynaecological use. With this instrument, the fibroid can be resected under direct vision. The resectoscope consists of a 26 French gauge outer sheath diameter and 0° or 30° fore-oblique telescope with a 4 mm outer diameter. All modern resectoscopes are of a continuous flow design, allowing constant turnover of distending media that facilitates visualization of the fibroid by rinsing out blood and debris. There is a large calibre inflow (cystoscopy tubing) and outflow tubing that are connected to a fluid management system. The inflow is pressurized with a peristaltic pump with a maximum pressure setting of 150 mmHg and a maximum flow setting of 450 mL/minute, similar to standard resectoscopy [42]. Pressures selected are based on the mean arterial pressure of the patient as a first-line barrier to fluid intravasation, typically 80 mmHg.

Standard technique to remove polyps and submucous myomas is resectoscopy with monopolar high-frequency electrical current. By means of a 5mm wire loop electrode, mounted on a working element with handpiece and integrated in an endoscope, tissue can be cut. Monopolar current necessitates the use of nonconducting, nonphysiologic, electrolyte-free irrigation and distention liquids such as sorbitol 5% or glycine 1.5% [3, 41, 42].

The outflow tubing should be connected to both the under the buttocks collection bag as well the outflow adaptor of the hysteroscope itself. This maintains a negative pressure in the outflow tract and allows for continuous suction of debris-laden fluid from the endometrial cavity and an accurate count of fluid lost. The negative pressure may be increased if the view is too cloudy or decreased if there is inadequate uterine distension prior to increasing the distension pressure [5, 41].

More commonly bipolar resectoscopes are being used as they require the use of isotonic conductive media, such as normal saline or lactate Ringers solution. This is because in a bipolar loop the active and return electrodes are in close proximity to one another a lower impedance media can be used. The risk of volume overload and electrolyte disturbance is significantly reduced with isotonic solutions.

Small-diameter bipolar electrodes or laser fibers can be passed through the instrument channel of most standard hysteroscope sheaths 5 mm or greater in diameter. In some instances, dissection of smaller submucous myomas can be accomplished with such energy sources.

The hysteroscopic morcellator is gaining more popularity in recent years. It was developed based on an orthopaedic shaver. It is a hollow device with a sideways opening that allows the blade to morcellate the leimyoma. It also has the ability to suction morcellated fragments of the fibroid simultaneously. This can also be used with saline distension media and does not require electrical current [42] (see **Figure 4**).

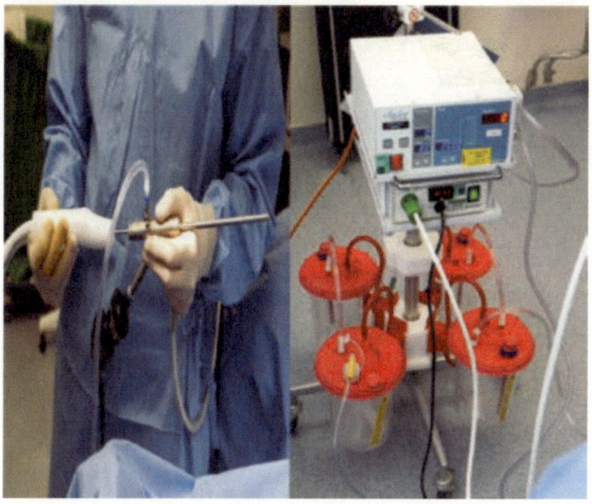

**Figure 4.** Surgeon holding *Myosure(Hologic)* hysteroscopic device (right). Inflow and outflow tubing for fluid management system (*Aquilex Hologic*) (left).

#### *4.2.2. Myomectomy procedure*

There are three basic methods for removing leiomyomas under hysteroscopic direction; morcellation, cutting with an electrosurgical loop and vaporization. The most commonly employed approaches use the resectoscope, a radiofrequency electrosurgical generator, and either a loop or a bulk-vapourising electrode.

When performing radiofrequency-based hysteroscopic myomectomy on women who wish to preserve fertility, care should be taken to minimize thermal damage to the tissue adjacent to the incision and that the loop does not touch adjacent healthy endometrium.

The traditional resectoscopic removal involves a slicing action of the fibroid. It can be performed with monopolar or bipolar cutting or coagulating current at a setting of 100 W. The electrosurgical loop is advanced beyond the fibroid and a repeated action of passing the cutting loop over the tissue in a backward direction, away from the fundus of the uterus is performed. In a pedunculated fibroid, the stalk can be transected and then removed by polyp forceps. Performing the procedure in a systematic way, starting at the top of the fibroid and working ones' way down to its base is the ideal approach. It is important to avoid damage to normal endometrial tissue with the loop as much as possible. Repetitively removing the resectoscope from the uterus to remove tissue fragments is time consuming, causes cervical trauma and can lead to a loss of uterine distention with compensatory increased use of distention media. To avoid this resected tissue, fragments can be pushed towards the uterine fundus and removed at the end of the operation. The closer the association of the fibroid with the serosa of the uterus, the more challenging the resection is due to the significant intramural component. Methods to facilitate extrusion of the intramural component include using the natural contractility of the uterus [43], intraoperative prostaglandins to stimulate uterine smooth muscle contraction [38], intravenous ergometrine [44] and repeated release of the uterine distending pressure, to allow for natural uterine extrusion.

For deep type 1 and type 2 fibroids that approach the uterine serosa (millimetres), it may be safer to perform a laparoscopy at the same time as the resection. This does not always prevent perforation but ensures early recognition of this complication and associated damage to other viscera. There is also the thought that the gas used to distend the abdominal cavity at laparoscopy can create a safety buffer in the unfortunate event of a perforation [45]. Type 0 and most type 1 fibroids are much more easily removed.

When a submucosal fibroid has a significant intramural component (type 2), a multi-staged procedure will result in a more complete resection and is generally also thought to be safer as it avoids the complication of perforation which can occur during resection of the base of the fibroid.

Electrosurgical vapourisation of fibroids involves using an electrode of cylindrical or spherical shape which uses current to vapourise the tissue. This does not produce any tissue fragments which can be a disadvantage if a specimen is required for histopathological assessment [46]. There is some lower quality evidence which suggests that reduced systemic absorption of distention media may occur with hysteroscopic myomectomy using this approach [47]. This could be because tissue fragments are not produced and the procedure can be performed faster without the need for removing tissue fragments. As with any current, the duration of contact, resistance of the tissue and the power (wattage) determine the degree of current delivered through the dispersive electrode. The surgeon is responsible for being aware of the power settings, as if they are too high there is a risk of skin burns to the patient through the skin plate (see **Figure 5**).

Another technique with increasing popularity is hysteroscopic morcellation. Using a modified prototype based on an orthopaedic arthroscopic tissue shaver, Dr. Mark Hans Emanuel was able to create a first-generation device that used mechanical energy rather than electrical energy to resect uterine tissue.

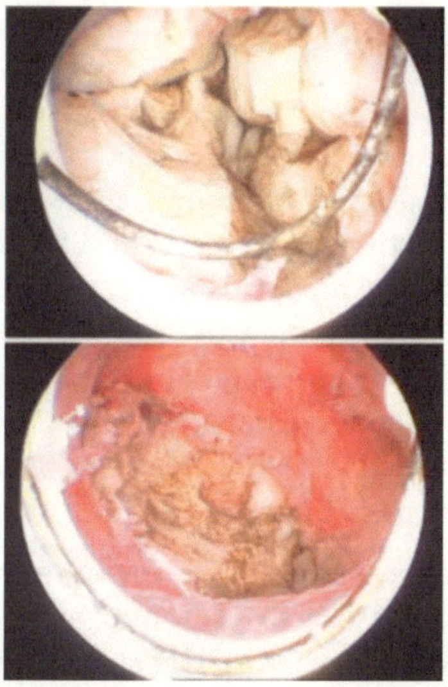

**Figure 5.** Hysteroscopic resection of a type 0 Fibroid (top) and at the end of a completed resection (bottom).

Hysteroscopic morcellation aims to remove uterine leiomyomas during a single insertion of a hysteroscope into the uterus. This contrasts with traditional hysteroscopic resection of leiomyomas, in which the instrument is reinserted into the uterus multiple times. Hysteroscopic morcellation is intended to reduce the risk of traumatic injury to the uterus and the risk of inadvertent fluid overload associated with traditional procedures (because the procedure may be completed more rapidly). An intended advantage of the procedure over thermal ablation techniques is avoiding the risk of thermal injury.

A hysteroscope is inserted into the uterus through the cervix, and saline is pumped through a small channel in the hysteroscope to distend the uterus. A specially designed morcellator is introduced via the hysteroscope and used to cut and simultaneously aspirate the leiomyoma tissue. The aspirated tissue can be collected for histological analysis. For polyps and type 0 and type 1 submucous myomas, hysteroscopic morcellation has been demonstrated to be both faster and easier to learn than traditional resectoscopy. The earliest published trial with a hysteroscopic morcellation device by Emanuel and colleagues showed a significant reduction in operating room time when removing polyps and type 0 and type 1 submucous myomas. In that study, polyps were removed with a 72% reduction in operating room time with a morcellator as compared with a resectoscope type 0 and type 1 myomas were removed in 61% less time, respectively [42]. Hence, hysteroscopic morcellation is most useful for small or pedunculated leiomyomas [48].

## 5. Complications

Hysteroscopic resection of submucosal fibroids is very safe in experienced hands. However, potential surgical complications include fluid overload, intraoperative and postoperative bleeding, uterine perforation, gas embolism, and infection with associated uterine synechiae.

### 5.1. Excessive fluid absorption

Excess absorption of non-crystalloid distension media can cause serious fluid and electrolyte imbalance, pulmonary and cerebral oedema, cardiac failure, and death [49]. Although complications associated with excess fluid absorption are relatively uncommonly encountered, premenopausal women undergoing resectoscopic surgery in the uterus may be at greater risk because of the inhibitory impact of female gonadal steroids (most likely estrogen) on the sodium/potassium ATP'ase pump [50]. Studies have demonstrated that 100 mL intravasation correlates with a sodium decrease of approximately 1 mmol/L. One study demonstrated that cerebral oedema could be identified during computed tomography scanning from an intravasation of only 500 mL. Therefore, a meticulous measure of the inflow and outflow of fluid used is extremely important [51].

Fluid absorption is increased when intrauterine pressure exceeds mean arterial pressure. Consequently, the intrauterine pressure should be maintained at the lowest pressure that allows good visualization for performance of the hysteroscopic myomectomy.

Nonconducting (electrolyte free) distention mediums such as glycine 1.5% or mannitol 5% are used with the monopolar electrosurgical system. With excess absorption of these fluids, there is a risk of hyponatraemia; however, the more serious complication is of cerebral oedema due to a hypo-osmolar effect on plasma concentration. This rare side effect can be fatal.

Electrolyte containing isotonic distention media (normal saline) can be used when mechanical or bipolar resections are employed. Its use reduces the risk of hyponatraemia and changes in serum osmolality when compared with nonconducting media. It can still cause fluid overload with consequent pulmonary oedema and therefore meticulous fluid balance should still be maintained.

### 5.2. Trauma

Other major complications consist of haemorrhage and uterine perforation. Perforation of the uterus can occur with dilators, mechanical grasping tools or the resectoscopic system. If perforation occurs with mechanical instruments, and no bowel injury is suspected, the patient can be managed expectantly with close observation for a 24-hour period. Laparoscopy must be performed if bowel injury is suspected, where there appears to be a large perforation, or in the presence of heavy bleeding. If perforation occurs with an activated electrode, one has to assume that there has been a bowel injury until proven otherwise, and laparoscopy or laparotomy is recommended.

Uterine perforation can be a complication with serious associated morbidity. Reassuringly, the risk of this is generally low. In a study of 2100 operative hysteroscopies performed by experienced surgeons, 782 involved fibroid resection and uterine perforation occurred in 1.2% of those procedures and 1.6% of all hysteroscopies [52]. The prospective Mistletoe study which analysed techniques of endometrial ablation demonstrated a slightly higher uterine perforation rate of up to 2.5% when using the electrosurgical resection loop [53]. Up to a third of uterine perforations are thought to occur during cervical dilatation before the resection is actually commenced. This could be avoided by use of cervical priming agents as discussed prior to allow easier dilatation. Unrecognized injury is a serious incident as it is possible that a bowel burn may have occurred, if perforation occurred when using an activated electrode, potentially leading to peritonitis and a high index of suspicion must always be exercised.

The above group also looked at rates of haemorrhage. Haemorrhage was defined as abnormal bleeding at the end of the procedure. In the 782 fibroid resections, the risk of operative haemorrhage was 0.4% [46].

### 5.3. Bleeding

Heavy bleeding from the endometrial cavity is uncommon after hysteroscopic surgery in general. If there is continuous bleeding after resection, a Foley catheter can be inserted into the uterine cavity and distended with up to 40 mL of saline until the bleeding settles from a tamponade effect. The balloon can be removed if the bleeding has settled in a few hours.

Other pharmacological agents that have been investigated to reduce blood loss at myomectomy include tranexamic acid, prostaglandin E2 analogues (misoprostol and dinoprostone) and ascorbic acid. Randomized controlled trails of these agents compared to placebo showed statistically significant reduction in blood loss; however, sample sizes in these studies were small and had low to moderate quality evidence [54].

A more invasive option for controlling bleeding is uterine artery embolization with interventional radiologic techniques if bleeding persists despite above measures.

### 5.4. Thermal burns

One must be very careful to avoid unintentional activation of the monopolar or bipolar pedals. If this occurs while the active electrode is resting on the patient it can cause serious burns to the abdomen, perineum, vagina or vulva [3].

More sinister burns occur when the uterus is perforated by an active electrode causing injury to surrounding structures, most commonly the bowel or blood vessels. This type of injury can be prevented by making sure not to activate the electrode while it is being advanced into the endometrial cavity. It should only be activated when being withdrawn. As discussed before, if a uterine perforation is suspected due to an active electrode, the surgeon must perform an exploratory laparoscopy or laparotomy depending on the extent of perforation.

### 5.5. Adhesions

Intrauterine adhesions can occur after hysteroscopic myomectomy to the point that they adversely impact fertility. The incidence of intrauterine adhesions after hysteroscopic myomectomy was shown in one study to be 7.5% [55]. Postoperative adjuvant therapy, including estrogen therapy for four to eight weeks or insertion of an intrauterine device, paediatric Foley catheter or other balloon for one week postoperatively, have all been used to prevent further adhesion development. However, there is scant evidence to support the use of these postoperative therapies [56, 57].

If, on preoperative assessment, it can be anticipated that a large proportion of the cavity will be stripped of endometrium after resection, an abdominal approach (laparotomy, laparoscopy or "robotic") to myomectomy should be considered to reduce the formation of adhesions. In a retrospective study, when second look hysteroscopy was performed after one to three months on 153 women who underwent TCRM, 2 of 132 (1.5%) with single myomectomy had intrauterine adhesions [58].

## 6. Effectiveness of hysteroscopic resection of submucosal fibroids

### 6.1. Management of subfertility

There is a lack of prospective randomized controlled trials assessing the true impact of surgical management of submucosal fibroids on fertility. This would be challenging to perform for obvious reasons. Many studies do not document that a comprehensive assessment of various causes of infertility was performed on the patient prior to surgery to isolate only those patients where the fibroid was the causative factor of subfertility. Other confounding factors are that conception rates are not recorded before and after surgery.

A recently published RCT compared TCRM with no treatment in 215 women with primary infertility with demonstrated submucous fibroids on ultrasound. The two randomized groups were women who underwent either TCRM or diagnostic hysteroscopy with biopsy only. At follow up, 63% of the treatment group conceived but only 28% of the biopsy group had (RR 2.1 CI 1.5–2.9). The investigators concluded that fertility rates increased after hysteroscopic myomectomy in women with type 0 and type 1 myomas ($p < 0.05$) but the same was not seen in women with type 2 myomas [59].

Similarly, Bozdag et al. demonstrated an improvement in spontaneous conception rates after the surgical removal of submucosal fibroids, but pregnancy rates following the removal of intramural or subserosal fibroids were no more improved than in the expectant management group of women with intramural or subserosal fibroids in situ [60]. A recent meta-analysis also demonstrated similar findings, with an improvement in pregnancy rates in infertile patients undergoing surgical removal of submucosal fibroids, but not in those undergoing surgical removal of intramural fibroids [27].

In summary, the evidence suggests that in women with otherwise unexplained infertility, submucosal fibroids should be removed in order to improve conception and pregnancy rates but removal of subserosal fibroids is not recommended, and this approach is endorsed by national bodies [61]. There is fair evidence to recommend against myomectomy in women with intramural fibroids (hysteroscopically confirmed intact endometrium) and otherwise unexplained infertility, regardless of the size of the fibroids.

### 6.2. Management of menorrhagia

Derman et al. in 1991 performed the first large-scale trial of the long-term success of hysteroscopic electrosurgical resection of fibroids [62]. Over a 9-year follow-up period, 84% of patients avoided a further procedure and 7% of patients needed a second hysteroscopic resection. Further studies by Emanuel et al. and Hart et al. showed that 91% of patients avoided further surgery at two years follow-up and 73% at eight years follow-up. It was also shown that risk factors for requiring surgery included a larger uterus and multiple fibroids [51].

Five series involving over 1400 women have shown that hysteroscopic myomectomy is an effective management option for dysfunctional uterine bleeding. Failure rates ranged from 14.5% to 30% for up to 4 years' follow-up [63]. This would suggest surgery should be considered as first-line treatment for the management of symptomatic fibroids, including submucous fibroids. Submucous myomas (types 0, 1 and 2) up to 5 cm in diameter can be removed hysteroscopically. Type 2 myomas are more likely to require a two-staged procedure than types 0 and 1 because of the risk of excessive fluid absorption and uterine perforation. The risk of uterine perforation is particularly high when there is less than 5 mm distance between the uterine serosa and the fibroid [2].

After TCRM alone, long-term cohort studies have indicated that patient satisfaction is in the range of 70–80%, with 14–16% of women requiring additional surgery [64].

When women with heavy menstrual bleeding who are not interested in future fertility and have selected type 2 and type 1 submucous myomas, generally 3 cm or less in diameter, endometrial ablation appears to confer a high degree of success in the short term [3]. In a single-armed, one-year study of the Novasure radiofrequency ablation system (Hologic Inc., Bedford, MA) in patients with type 1 or 2 myomas, 95% of the 65 patients were successfully treated [65]. At the present time, there is inadequate evidence to suggest that one device or technique, such as resectoscopic ablation, is clearly more efficacious than another.

Therefore, if the main symptom is heavy menstrual bleeding only and fertility is not required, consideration should be given at the time of transcervical resection of myoma to also perform endometrial ablation. This has been demonstrated in a cohort study, which showed a higher success rate in controlling bleeding when ablation was added to myomectomy [66].

## 7. Repeat resection of fibroids

As can be seen from the success of surgery, for most patients the chance of avoiding further surgery is about 80% with long-term follow-up [67], but the success is lower in patients with type 2 fibroids [2, 67].

The recurrence rate of fibroids is 15% and 10% of women who have a myomectomy will eventually need a hysterectomy within 10 years. Factors more likely to be associated with recurrence of fibroids are the woman's age, number of fibroids, larger uterine size and childbirth after myomectomy [68].

The success rate of a repeat resection has been described by Istre and Langebrekke [17]. Twenty-eight per cent of their 118 patients who needed repeat surgery (ablation or myomectomy) eventually proceeded to a hysterectomy. The main indication was pain due to a haematometra. One of the major causes of primary surgery failure was found to be deep adenomyosis and associated pain. It was suggested that MRI could be used as a diagnostic tool in those presenting with failed initial surgery, to select patients with adenomyosis, who are less likely to benefit from repeat surgery unless it is a hysterectomy. Of course, this option would not be of use to patients wishing to preserve fertility [69].

## Acknowledgements

We would like to thank the authors of the publications cited who have enabled us to write an up-to-date account of hysteroscopic surgery of submucosal fibroids. We would like to recognize these two publications as providing some of the background to our chapter, *'The hysteroscopic management of leiomyomata by Prof R Hart in Uterine Leiomyomas: Pathogenesis and Management'* and the *'AAGL practice report: practice guidelines for the diagnosis and management of submucous leiomyomas in the Journal of Minimally Invasive Gynecology.'*

## Author details

Rashi Kalra[1,2] and Roger J Hart[2,3*]

*Address all correspondence to: roger.hart@uwa.edu.au

1 King Edward Memorial Hospital, Subiaco, Perth, Australia

2 Fertility Specialists of Western Australia, Bethesda Hospital, Claremont, WA, Australia

3 School of Women's and Infants' Health, King Edward Memorial Hospital, University of Western Australia, Perth, WA, Australia

## References

[1] EE Wallach, NF Vlahos. Uterine myomas: an overview of development, clinical features, and management. Obstet Gynecol. 2004;104:393–406.

[2] K Wamsteker, S DeBlok, A Galilnat, RP Lueken. Transcervical hysteroscopic resection of submucous fibroids for abnormal uterine bleeding: results regarding the degree of intramural extension. Obstet Gynecol. 1993;82:736–40.

[3] J Abbott, MG Munro, L Muzzi. AAGL practice report: practice guidelines for the diagnosis and management of submucous leiomyomas. J Minim Invasive Gynecol.. 2012;19(2):152–71.

[4] MH Emanuel, K Wamsteker, AA Hart, G Metz. Long-term results of hysteroscopic myomectomy for abnormal uterine bleeding. Obstet Gynecol. 1999;93:743–48.

[5] Hart, Roger. The Hysteroscopic Management of Fibroids. In: Brosens I, editor. Uterine Leiomyomas: Pathogenesis and Management: Taylor and Francis Medical Books, Oxfordshire, UK, 2005.

[6] P Vercellini, I Cortesi, S Oldani, et al. The role of transvaginal ultrasonography and outpatient diagnostic hysteroscopy in the evaluation of women with menorrhagia. Hum Reprod. 1997;12:1768–71.

[7] FA Van den Brule, O Wery, J Huveneers, UJ Gaspard. Comparison of contrast hysterosonography and transvaginal ultrasonography for uterus imaging. J Gynecol Obstet Biol Reprod. 1999;28:131–6.

[8] C Farquhar, A Ekeroma, S Furness, B Arroll. A systematic review of transvaginal ultrasonography, sonohysterography and hysteroscopy for the investigation of abnormal uterine bleeding in premenopausal women. Acta Obstet Gynecol Scand. 2003;82:493–504.

[9] M Ruach, R Hart, A Magos. Outpatient hysteroscopy. Contemp Rev Obstet Gynaecol. 1998;10:295–302.

[10] MJ Cooper, JA Broadbent, BG Molnar et al. A series of 1000 consecutive out-patient diagnostic hysteroscopies. J Obstet Gynaecol. 1995;21:503–7.

[11] F Nagele, G Lockwood, AL Magos. Randomised placebo controlled trial of mefenamic acid for premedication at outpatient hysteroscopy: a pilot study. Br J Obstet Gynaecol. 1997;104:842–4.

[12] F Nagele, N Bournas, H O'Connor H, et al. Comparison of carbon dioxide and normal saline for uterine distension in outpatient hysteroscopy. Fertil Steril. 1996;65:305–9.

[13] CP Stamatopoulos, T Mikos, GF Grimbizis, AS Dimitriadis, I Efstratiou, P Stamatopoulos, et al. Value of magnetic resonance imaging in diagnosis of adenomyosis and myomas of the uterus. J Minim Invasive Gynecol. 2012;19:620–26.

[14] M Dueholm, E Lundorf, ES Hansen, S Ledertoug, F Olesen. Accuracy of magnetic resonance imaging and transvaginal ultrasonography in the diagnosis, mapping, and measurement of uterine myomas. Am J Obstet Gynecol. 2002;186:409–15.

[15] M Dueholm, E Lundorf, ES Hansen, S Ledertoug, F Olesen. Evaluation of the uterine cavity with magnetic resonance imaging, transvaginal sonography, hysterosonographic examination and diagnostic hysteroscopy. Fertil Steril. 2001;76:350–57 (II–1).

[16] BJ Vollenhoven, AS Lawrence, DL Healy. Uterine fibroids: a clinical review. Br J Obstet Gynaecol. 1990;97:285.

[17] O Istre. A Langebrekke Repeat hysteroscopic surgery reduces the hysterectomy rate after endometrial and myoma resection. J Am Assoc Gynecol Laparosc. 2003;10:247–51.

[18] MG Munro, HO Critchley, MS Broder, IS Fraser. The FIGO Classification System ("PALM-COEIN") for causes of abnormal uterine bleeding in non-gravid women in the reproductive years, including guidelines for clinical investigation. Int J Gynaecol Obstet. 2011(113);1:3–13.

[19] C Farquhar, B Arroll, A Ekeroma, G Fentiman et al. An evidence-based guideline for the management of uterine fibroids. New Zealand Guidelines Group 2000.

[20] JA Broadbent, AL Magos. Menstrual blood loss after hysteroscopic myomectomy. Gynae Endosc. 1995;4:41–4.

[21] MA Lumsden, EM Wallace. Clinical presentation of uterine fibroids. Baillieres Clin Obstet Gynaecol. 1998;12:177–95.

[22] T Eldar-Geva, S Meagher, DL Healy, V MacLachlan, S Breheny, C Wood. Effect of intramural, subserosal, and submucosal uterine fibroids on the outcome of assisted reproductive technology treatment. Fertil Steril. 1998;70:687–91.

[23] J Farhi, J Ashkenazi, D Feldberg, D Dicker, R Orvieto, Z Ben Rafael. Effect of uterine leiomyomata on the results of in-vitro fertilization treatment. Hum Reprod. 1995;10: 2576–8.

[24] B Carranza-Mamane, Jon Havelock, R Hemmings et al. The management of uterine fibroids in women with otherwise unexplained infertility. J Obstet Gynaecol Can. 2015;37(3):277–85.

[25] J Donnez, P Jadoul. What are the implications of myomas on fertility? A need for a debate? Hum Reprod. 2002;17:424–30.

[26] EA Pritts. Fibroids and infertility: a systematic review of the evidence. Obstet Gynecol Surv. 2001;56:483–91.

[27] EA Pritts, WH Parker, DL Olive. Fibroids and infertility: an updated systematic review of the evidence. Fertil Steril. 2009;91:1215–23.

[28] Guidelines, RANZCOG. Fibroids in infertility. Royal Australian and New Zealand College of Obstetricians and Gynaecologists, 2014.

[29] RS Neuwirth, HK Amin HK. Excision of submucous fibroids with hysteroscopic control. Am J Obstet Gynecol. 1976;126(III):95–9.

[30] RB Lasmar, PR Barrozo, R Dias, MA Oliveira. Submucous myomas: a new presurgical classification to evaluate the viability of hysteroscopic surgical treatment–preliminary report. J Minim Invasive Gynecol. 2005;12(II–2):308–11.

[31] P Vercellini, B Zaina, L Yaylayan, A Pisacreta, O De Giorgi, PG Crosignani. Hysteroscopic myomectomy: long-term effects on menstrual pattern and fertility. Obstet Gynecol. 1999;94:341–347 (II–2).

[32] T Shokeir, M El-Shafei, H Yousef, AF Allam, E Sadek. Submucous myomas and their implications in the pregnancy rates of patients with otherwise unexplained primary infertility undergoing hysteroscopic myomectomy: a randomized matched control study. Fertil Steril. 2010;94(I):724–29.

[33] GA Vilos, C Allaire, PY Laberge, N Leyland, et al. The management of uterine leiomyomas. J Obstet Gynaecol Can. 2015;37(2):157–78.

[34] TG Stovall, FW Ling, LC Henry, MR Woodruff. A randomized trial evaluating leuprolide acetate before hysterectomy as treatment for leiomyomas. Am J Obstet Gynecol. 1991;164:1420–3.

[35] R Garry, A Khair, P Mooney, M Stuart. A comparison of goserelin and danazol as endometrial thinning agents prior to endometrial laser ablation. Br J Obstet Gynaecol. 1996;103:339–44.

[36] T Kalampokas, M Kamath, I Boutas, E Kalampokas. Ulipristal acetate for uterine fibroids: a systematic review and meta-analysis. Gynecol Endocrinol. 2016;32(2):91–6.

[37] C Batukan, MT Ozgun, B Ozcelik, E Aygen, Y Sahin, C Turkyilmaz. Cervical ripening before operative hysteroscopy in premenopausal women: a randomized, double-blind, placebo-controlled comparison of vaginal and oral misoprostol. Fertil Steril. 2008;89(I): 966–73.

[38] VM McCausland, GA Fields, AM McCausland, DE Townsend. Tuboovarian abscesses after operative hysteroscopy. J Reprod Med. 1993;38(III):198–200.

[39] AL Magos, R Baumann, GM Lockwood, AC Turnbull. Experience with the first 250 endometrial resections for menorrhagia. Lancet. 1991;337:1074–8.

[40] Patrick Mcilwaine, Bernadette Mcelhinney, Krishnan Andrew Karthigasu, Roger Hart. A prospective study of the use of the Myosure resectoscope to manage endometrial polyps in an outpatient setting. Aust N Z J Obstet Gynaecol. 2015;55:482–7.

[41] MJ Solnik, R Azziz, Hysteroscopic Myomectomy In: Gaertner R, editor. Te Linde's Atlas of Gynaecologic Surgery. Philadelphia, PA, USA: Lippincott Williams & Wilkins, 2014. p. 231–39.

[42] Mark Emanuel, Kees Wamsteker. The intra uterine morcellator: a new hysteroscopic operating technique to remove intrauterine polyps and myomas. J Minim Invasive Gynecol. 2005;12(1):62–6.

[43] FD Loffer. Removal of large symptomatic intrauterine growths by the hysteroscopic resectoscope. Obstet Gynecol. 1990;76(5 Pt 1):836–40.

[44] A Darwish, A Darwish. Modified hysteroscopic myomectomy of large submucous fibroids. Gynecol Obstet Invest 2003;56:192–6.

[45] L Mencaglia, E Tiso, R Bianchi, C Tantini. Intramural Myomectomy Using a combination of hysteroscopy and laparoscopy. J Am Assoc Gynecol Laparosc. 1996;3(Suppl): S30.

[46] PG Brooks. Resectoscopic myoma vaporizer. J Reprod Med. 1995;40(III):791–95.

[47] P Vercellini, S Oldani, O DeGiorgi, II Cortesi, M Moschetta, PG Crosignani. Endometrial ablation with a vaporizing electrode in women with regular uterine cavity or submucous leiomyomas. J Am Assoc Gynecol Laparosc. 1996;3(II–2):S52.

[48] Guidelines, NICE. Hysteroscopic morcellation of uterine leiomyomas (fifibroids). 2015 Contract No.: IPG522.

[49] O Istre, J Bjoennes, R Naess, K Hornbaek, A Forman. Postoperative cerebral oedema after transcervical endometrial resection and uterine irrigation with 1.5% glycine. Lancet. 1994;344(II–2):1187–9.

[50] O Taskin, A Buhur, M Birincioglu, F Burak, R Atmaca, I Yilmaz, et al. Endometrial Na1, K1-ATPase pump function and vasopressin levels during hysteroscopic surgery in patients pretreated with GnRH agonist. J Am Assoc Gynecol Laparosc. 1998;5(I):119–24.

[51] MH Emanuel, AAM Hart, K Wamsteker, et al. An analysis of fluid-loss during transcervical resection of submucous myomas. Fertil Steril. 1997;68:881–6.

[52] Agostini A, Cravello L, Bretelle F, Shojai R, Roger V, Blanc B. Risk of uterine perforation during hysteroscopic surgery. J Am Assoc Gynecol Laparosc. 2002;9:264–7.

[53] C Overton, J Hargreaves, M Maresh. A national survey of the complications of endometrial destruction for menstrual disorders: the MISTLETOE study. Br J Obstet Gynaecol 1997;104:1351–9.

[54] EJ Kongnyuy, CS Wiysonge. Interventions to reduce haemorrhage during myomectomy for fibroids (Review). The Cochrane Library 2015(8):CD005355.

[55] C Touboul, H Fernandez, X Deffieux, R Berry, R Frydman, A Gervaise. Uternine syndechiae after bipolar hysteroscopic resection of submucosal myomas in patients with infertility. Fertil Steril. 2009;92:1690–3.

[56] PH Kodaman, A Arici A. Intrauterine adhesions and fertility outcome: how to optimize success? Curr Opin Obstet Gynecol. 2007;19:207–14.

[57] EA Tonguc, T Var, N Yilmaz, S Batioglu. Intrauterine device or estrogen treatment after hysteroscopic septum resection. Int J Gynaecol Obstet. 2010;109:226–9.

[58] JH Yang, MJ Chen, MY Wu, KH Chao, HN Ho, YS Yang. Office hysteroscopic early lysis of intrauterine adhesion after transcervical resection of multiple apposing submucous myomas. Fertil Steril. 2008;89(II–2):1254–9.

[59] T Shokeir, M El-Shafei, H Yousef, AF Allam, E Sadek. Submucous myomas and their implications in the pregnancy rates of patients with otherwise unexplained primary infertility undergoing hysteroscopic myomectomy: a randomized matched control study. Fertil Steril. 2010;94:724–729 (I). Fertil Steril. 2010;94(I):724–29.

[60] G Bozdag, I Esinler, K Boynukalin, T Aksu, S Gunalp, T Gurgan Single intramural leiomyoma with normal hysteroscopic findings does not affect ICSI-embryo transfer outcome. Reprod Biomed Online. 2009;19:276–80.

[61] B Kroon, N Johnson, M Chapman, A Yazdani, R Hart. Fibroids in infertility—consensus statement from ACCEPT (Australasian CREI Consensus Expert Panel on Trial evidence). Australasian CREI Consensus Expert Panel on Trial evidence (ACCEPT) group. Aust N Z J Obstet Gynaecol. 2011;51(4):289–95.

[62] SG Derman, J Rehnstrom, RS Neuwirth. The long-term effectiveness of hysteroscopic treatment of menorrhagia and leiomyomas. Obstet Gynecol. 1991;77:591–4.

[63] Munro, MG. Abnormal uterine bleeding: surgical management—part 3. J Am Assoc Gynecol Laparosc. 2001;8:818–47.

[64] V Polena, JL Mergui, N Perrot, C Poncelet, E Barranger, S Uzan. Long-term results of hysteroscopic myomectomy in 235 patients. Eur J Obstet Gynecol Reprod Biol. 2007;30(II–2):232–7.

[65] R Sabbah, G Desaulniers Use of the NovaSure Impedance Controlled Endometrial Ablation System in patients with intracavitary disease: 12-month follow-up results of a prospective, single-arm clinical study. J Minim Invasive Gynecol. 2006;13(II–2):467–71.

[66] Loffer, FD. Improving results of hysteroscopic submucousal myomectomy for menorrhagia by concomitant endometrial ablation. J Minim Invasive Gynecol. 2005;12:254–60.

[67] R Hart, BG Molnar, A Magos. Long term follow up of hysteroscopic myomectomy assessed by survival analysis. Br J Obstet Gynaecol. 1999;106:700–5.

[68] Garcia, CR. Management of the symptomatic fibroid in women older than 40 years of age: hysterectomy or myomectomy? Obstet Gynecol Clin North Am. 1993;20:337–48.

[69] R Hart, A Magos. Endometrial ablation. Curr Opin Obstet Gynecol. 1997;9:226–32.

Section 3

# Fertility-oriented Laparoscopic Surgery

Chapter 3

# Endometriosis: When and How We Treat

Sidonia Maria Saceanu, Stefan Patrascu,

Anca Patrascu and Valeriu Surlin

Additional information is available at the end of the chapter

http://dx.doi.org/10.5772/65296

**Abstract**

Endometriosis is a chronic, nonmalignant and estrogen-dependent disease in which endometrial glandular epithelium and stroma are outside the uterine cavity (ovaries, peritoneum, or rectovaginal septum). The prevalence is estimated from 2 to 10% in women of childbearing age and it rises up to 50% in women with infertility. Despite maximal efforts, the therapy of first choice in the management of endometriosis is still unclear. The aim of this chapter is to present an update of its management, emphasizing the benefits and disadvantages of surgical methods. We performed a systematic literature search on the PubMed database of English literature (search terms: endometrioma, surgery, ovarian reserve, assisted reproductive technologies) from 2010 to 2014. For endometrioma, operative laparoscopy proved to be the gold standard. Surgical procedures consist of partial excision of the cyst wall and electro-coagulation of the rest. Stripping technique may be a better method for reducing the recurrence of pain symptoms, recurrence, and reoperation rates, but it raises concerns about ovarian reserve. For endometriosis, surgery often includes partial rectum or sacrouterine ligament resection. Hysterectomy is not obligatory and refused by the young patients. The approach should be laparoscopic and if necessary vaginal assisted. Good cooperation between various disciplines (gynecology, surgery, urology) is mandatory.

**Keywords:** endometriosis, endometrioma, laparoscopy, ovarian reserve, fertility

# 1. Introduction

## 1.1. Definitions

Endometriosis is a chronic, nonmalignant, and estrogen-dependent disease in which the endometrial glandular epithelium and stroma are found outside the uterine cavity (on the ovaries, peritoneum, or rectovaginal septum) [1].

The most frequently type of endometriosis is endometrioma. Concretely, an endometrioma is considered as the presence of endometrial tissue at the ovarian level organized as a cyst [2]. The incidence of endometrioma is estimated to be 20–45% of patients with endometriosis [3]. It can be diagnosed by ultrasound with relatively high sensitivity of 74%, but with a very high specificity of 94%; therefore, its prevalence could be estimated quite precisely [1, 4].

Although endometriosis usually affects ovaries and peritoneum, deep endometriosis, defined as infiltration of the peritoneum by a minimum of 5 mm can affect other structures like urinary tract, fallopian tubes, and bowels [1, 3].

Compared to ovarian endometriosis, very little is known about deeply infiltrating endometriosis. In this form, endometriosis can spread beyond organ borders and infiltrate various structures like sacrouterine ligament, the rectovaginal septum, the fornix of the vagina, the rectosigmoid, the urinary bladder or the ureter or also the small intestine [1–5].

## 1.2. Epidemiology

Despite its severity, endometriosis is a common benign gynecological disease [6].

The prevalence of endometriosis is estimated to range from 2 to 10% in women of childbearing age and its prevalence rises up to 50% in women with infertility [7]. It is one of the most common gynecological problems that can affect women in their reproductive years [4].

## 1.3. Pathogenesis

Endometriosis is a complex and multifactorial disease and its etiology and pathogenesis have not yet been completely clarified [8].

Many authors have described a group of risk factors like retrograde menstruation caused by the obstruction of menstrual flow, low immunity, exposure to diethylstilbestrol during neonatal period, genetic predisposition [2–4]. Another theory suggests that endometrial tissue is distributed from the uterus to other parts of the body through the lymph system or blood system [5–8]. Surgical implants have also been cited in many cases where endometriosis is found in abdominal laparotomy scars, like after a cesarean section [9, 10].

Other authors suggest that risk factors for endometriosis are smoking, duration of period bleeding, length of the menstrual cycle, number of pregnancies, and number of miscarriages [3–9].

In endometriosis, the ectopic endometrial tissue is morphologically similar to normal endometrium and it responds to ovarian hormones during cyclical changes similar to eutopic endometrium [11].

### 1.4. Diagnosis and evolution

Women with endometriosis may be asymptomatic, but the majority will present with pelvic pain, adnexal mass or subfertility/ infertility [3].

Definitive diagnosis is made through direct operative visualization by laparoscopy (**Figure 1**) or laparotomy and histological confirmation [9].

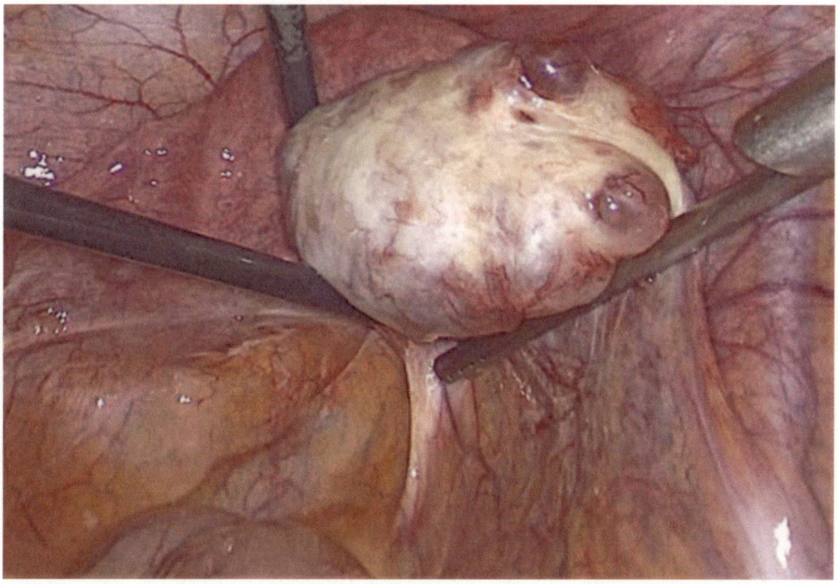

**Figure 1.** Twenty-four years old female patient, complaining of severe menstrual pain, with large endometrioma of the right ovary (5 cm).

On laparoscopy, endometriosis can appear as yellow-brown discolorations, raised flame-like patches, whitish opacifications or reddish irregularly shaped spots [1, 2].

Patients with endometriosis may present different clinical manifestations in different stages of the disease [10].

Endometriosis has four stages or types: stage I, minimal, with small lesions and shallow endometrial implants on the ovary; stage 2, mild, with light lesions and shallow implants on the ovary and the pelvic lining; stage 3, moderate, with deep and more implants on the ovary and pelvic lining; and stage 4, severe, with deep implants on the pelvic lining and ovaries [1–11].

Ovarian endometriomas, which are a common feature of endometriosis, create a complex situation for infertile patients [5].

In the opinion of many authors, endometriosis is one of the top three causes of female infertility and 30% to 40 % of women with endometriosis are infertile [5–6].

Fadhlaoui et al. showed that women with endometriosis have a reduced monthly fecundity rate (2–10%) compared with fertile couples (15–20%) at the same age [11]. The mechanisms underlying reproductive failure remain controversial, especially in cases where ovaries and fallopian tubes are normal [7].

The mechanism by which these endometriotic cysts lead to infertility may be related to mechanical stretching of the ovarian cortex as well as an inflammatory reaction with cytotoxic oxidative stress and increased fibrosis [1–3]. Surgery is the elective treatment for endometriomas and the most common technique is stripping of the endometrioma [11].

Both the presence and surgical excision of endometriomas appear to be damaging to ovarian function and ovarian reserve [6].

## 2. Treatment of endometriosis

### 2.1. Methods

We made a systematic literature search on the PubMed database of English literature (search terms was endometrioma, surgery, ovarian reserve, assisted reproductive technologies) from 2010 to 2014 and cross referencing. We gave priority to meta-analyses, randomized controlled trials reviews and cohort studies. We analyzed the benefits and disadvantages of surgical methods used to treat endometriosis.

### 2.2. Results

The treatment of endometriosis depends on the age of the patient, extent of disease, severity of symptom and the desired outcomes for fertility [1]. Despite maximal efforts, the therapy of first choice in the management of endometriosis is still unclear [12, 13].

#### *2.2.1. Medical versus surgical therapy*

Because endometriosis is a chronic disease, medical therapy should be, at least in theory, the first choice of treatment, while surgical procedures should be reserved for patients who do not respond to conservative treatments and whose symptoms affect their quality of life or cause infertility [8].

The aim of medical therapy is to achieve a hypoestrogenic status or to induce a pseudopregnancy [9]. Endometriosis implants can be regressively changed by means of suppression of ovarian function [11]. The drugs predominately used today are pure gestagens, progestatives, contraceptives, GnRH analogs, and danazol [5–7].

Every medical treatment is tolerable but should only be used as long as it is necessary [12]. This type of treatment should reduce the number of surgical interventions and improve the quality of life [13, 14].

Medical therapy can be also applied prior to surgery to decrease the size of endometriotic implants and the extent of the operation [1].

Another method consists of a combination of diagnostic laparoscopy with the removing of all visible endometriosis as far as possible followed by 3–6 months of endocrine therapy and a subsequent second-look laparoscopy with resection of residual foci, adhesiolysis, and reconstruction of organs [10–14].

So far there is no evidence that perioperative or postoperative hormonal treatment delays or prevents recurrence, reduce pelvic pain and patient's morbidity or increases pregnancy rates at a statistically significant level [15].

### 2.2.2. *Rationale for surgery*

Because endometriosis is a progressive and evolutive disease, which can cause anatomic destruction of the reproductive organs and infertility, surgical therapy has an important role [6–10].

The surgical treatment for endometriosis can be conservative or radical. The benefit of surgical treatment is to reduce or reverse the damaging effects of endometriomas on the ovarian cortex, but this effect is controversial [14]. Surgery's aim is to remove macroscopic endometriosis implants, the adhesions, and restore normal pelvic anatomy [10].

Evidence indicates that the primary benefit of surgical treatment of endometriosis is relief of pelvic pain [7–10].

Another argument in favor of surgical excision of endometriomas is related to the dangers of expected management, such as ovarian torsion, cyst rupture, and progression of endometriosis [6–10]. The risk of ovarian malignancy is debatable, as some authors reported that endometriosis can be associated with increased risk of clear cell ovarian cancer or low-grade serous ovarian cancer [3]. Future research should be focused on understanding the mechanisms that might lead to malignant transformation of endometriosis to help identify the women at risk [4].

### 2.2.3. *Objectives of surgery*

As it was mentioned before, surgical treatment may be conservative or radical.

The goal of conservative surgery is to remove or destroy endometrial abnormal proliferation without damaging the reproductive organs [8].

Radical surgery for endometriosis aims to eliminate all possible endometriosis implants found in pelvic and abdominal cavity, including hysterectomy and bilateral adnexectomy, and to excise of the deep endometriosis lesions that can involve the urinary and digestive organs, as well as the rectovaginal and/or vesicouterine space. However, this technique has to be of last resort because it is radical and definitive [16–19].

*2.2.4. Laparoscopic versus open approach*

Surgery can be done through open surgery or by laparoscopy [10]. Minimally invasive techniques were proved to be feasible in treating endometriosis [14].

Many studies including two randomized controlled trials, comparing medical treatment with laparoscopic excision of endometrioma concluded that laparoscopic excision is associated with a decrease in symptoms such as dysmenorrhea, dyspareunia, and nonmenstrual pelvic pain [10–15].

Compared to laparotomy, operative laparoscopy was proved to be the gold standard surgical approach for the diagnosis and treatment of endometriosis [12].

Concerning the open access, the decision to use this type of access is very important. It is recommended that laparotomy should be performed only in cases with massive endometriosis, in older patients or in cases where pelvic pain and discomfort are the main problems for the patients [10–15]. The selection should be done, because this type of treatment obviously takes longer operative time is more painful and it involves a longer hospital stay. The risks and side effects are also greater than for laparoscopy. It is therefore better to almost never use laparotomy as a treatment for endometriosis [14]. Therefore, laparotomy should only be reserved to very difficult cases.

Laparoscopy is a central component in the diagnosis of and therapy for endometriosis. Laparoscopy is initially used to diagnose endometriosis. Visualization of areas of endometriosis may be followed by excision or destruction by burning (**Figure 2**). This can be done simply with the diathermy or using the laser. However, the laser is expensive, time-consuming, and almost never used now by leading endometriosis surgeons [10–12].

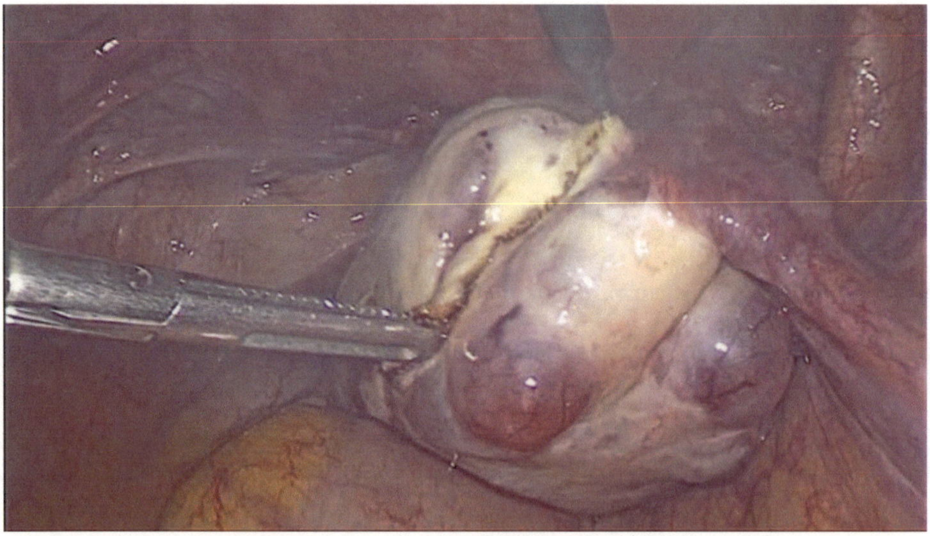

**Figure 2.** Laparoscopic incision of an endometriotic cyst of the ovary using diathermy.

Conventional laparoscopy has several proven advantages over laparotomy, like faster postoperative recovery, shorter length of hospital stay, cosmetic benefits, decreased blood loss, and fewer complications [16, 17]. However, laparoscopic management of advanced-stage endometriosis requires pelvic dissection, which can increase the surgeon fatigue, operating time, rate of conversion to laparotomy, intraoperative, and postoperative complications [18].

Robotic-assisted laparoscopic surgery tries to overcome the disadvantages of conventional laparoscopy by offering improved dexterity, better coordination, and visualization of organs and less surgeon fatigue [19].

Many studies acknowledge that laparoscopy is especially indicated for patients with moderate or severe endometriosis or for those who accuse pain or infertility [4].

The risk factors and disadvantages of laparoscopy include damage of organs adjacent to the affected areas and postoperative complications, such as adhesion formation or infection [8].

Some authors emphasized that the management of an endometrioma must focus on the complex pathology of this disease further confirming through ovarioscopy biopsies that endometriomas *in situ* have progressive smooth muscle cell metaplasia and fibrosis of the cortical layer. Additionally, they found no correlation between the size of the endometrioma and the degree of ovarian pathology [10–16].

Recently, in several studies, a new approach called transvaginal hydrolaparoscopy is mentioned. By this approach, an endometrioma could be confirmed by its appearance in gross anatomy and even removed in an early stage [8–12]. Transvaginal ovarioscopy, associated or not with ablation, is performed in numerous medical centers [15–18] and could be considered a variant of NOTES (natural orifice tranlumenal endoscopic surgery).

*2.2.5. Laparoscopic procedures*

The surgical procedures that can be performed during an operative laparoscopy usually include the excision or destruction of ovarian endometriosis (endometriomas) (**Figure 3**), the removal or destruction of endometrial implants, adhesiolysis, oophorectomy, hysterectomy, the removal of deep rectovaginal and rectosigmoid endometriosis, surgery of the bowel (usually enterectomy) or bladder, laparoscopic uterine nerve ablation (LUNA), and presacral neurectomy (PSN) [1–8].

Although the ovarian endometrioma is described as an ovarian cyst, its pathology is rather complex and completely different from other benign ovarian cysts [18–20]. According to Huhesdon, the majority of endometriomas are thought to be pseudocysts rather than intraovarian cysts, as the clear dissection plane between an endometrioma and ovarian cortex may not always exist, like in other benign ovarian cysts [19, 20].

While most endometrial implants can be treated using excision or/and coagulation, the most frequently used surgical procedures for the treatment of ovarian endometriosis are the excision of the cyst capsula or electro-coagulation of the cyst wall (**Figure 4**) [7–10]. During excision, the endometrioma is aspirated followed by the removal of the cyst wall from the ovary cortex. However, this technique could reduce ovarian reserve and decrease the chances of fertility [10–14]. Concerning this last aspect, there is currently no randomized controlled trial to assess whether surgery is positively effective or not on pregnancy rates in moderate to severe endometriosis [19]. However, there are numerous nonrandomized uncontrolled studies with results indicating a postoperative pregnancy rate that varies widely from 30 to 67% [19–21].

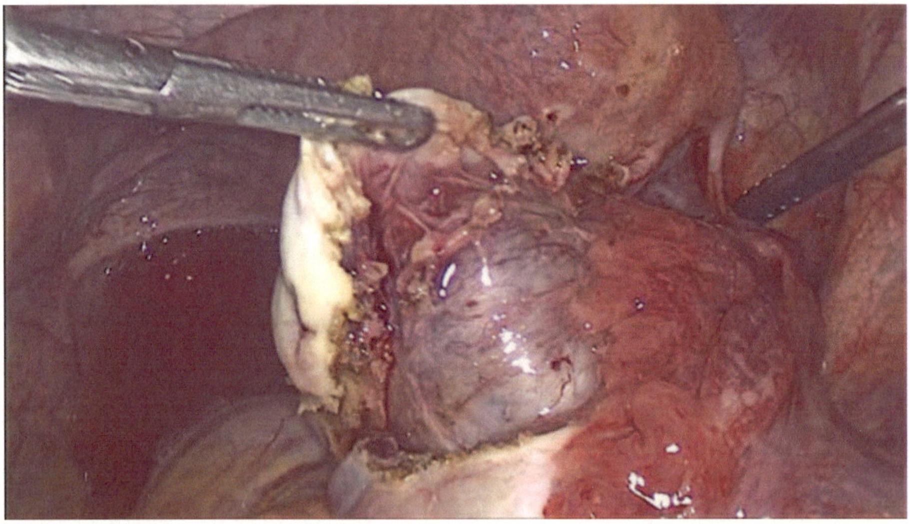

**Figure 3.** Excision of an endometrioma: cleavage plane between the endometrioma and ovary, progressive dissection through divergent traction.

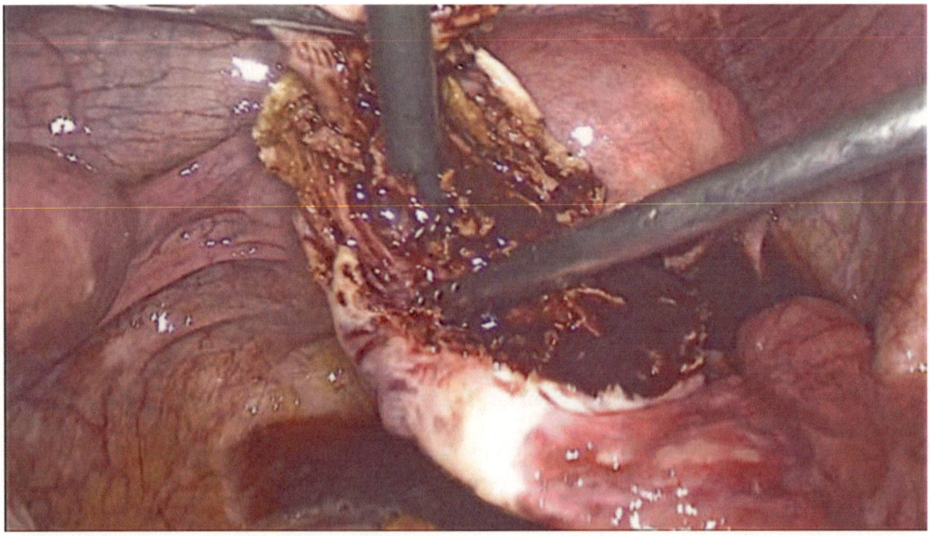

**Figure 4.** Enucleation of endometrioma of the right ovary.

The recommendations of the ESHRE guidelines for women with endometriomas who are undergoing surgery for infertility or pain, strongly support the laparoscopic excision rather than drainage and electrocoagulation of the endometrioma wall [21–23]. Several studies showed that the stripping technique is superior to drainage or ablative surgery because it reduces the recurrence of pain, and it is decreasing the recurrence and reoperation rates [18, 19].

According to the ESHRE Guideline, in infertile women with ovarian endometrioma bigger than 3 cm surgeons should perform excision of endometrioma capsule instead of ablative surgery because the studies show that it increases the spontaneous postoperative pregnancy rate (**Figure 5**) [20–23].

Technique of laparoscopic removal of endometrioma begins by incision of the ovary and finding the dissection plane between the endometrial cyst and the ovarian parenchyma. Dissection may progress carefully and slowly in this fashion until its completion. However, to facilitate dissection the cyst may be opened, its content evacuated by aspiration, and the walls of the cyst literally stripped away by divergent traction (traction and counter-traction) from the ovarian parenchyma. This is a commonly used technique [20–22]. In our opinion, evacuation of the cyst's contents should be performed carefully and complete, and at the end, the pelvic cavity immediately and thoroughly washed with saline or iodine–povidone solution to prevent iatrogenic spreading of endometriosis. The remaining ovarian parenchyma is coagulated by bipolar or monopolar cautery and could be left open or could be sutured [23]. We prefer to leave it open to allow drainage and avoid formation of intraovarian hematic collections that could lead to ovarian abscesses. Another possibility of surgical treatment is to electrocoagulate by diathermy or by laser energy the inner cavity of the cyst after evacuation instead of removing it [1, 4]. We consider that if the dissection is not amenable or hemostasis is difficult, those two methods could be combined in the sense that a part of the cyst wall could be left in the place but its inner surface coagulated as mentioned before.

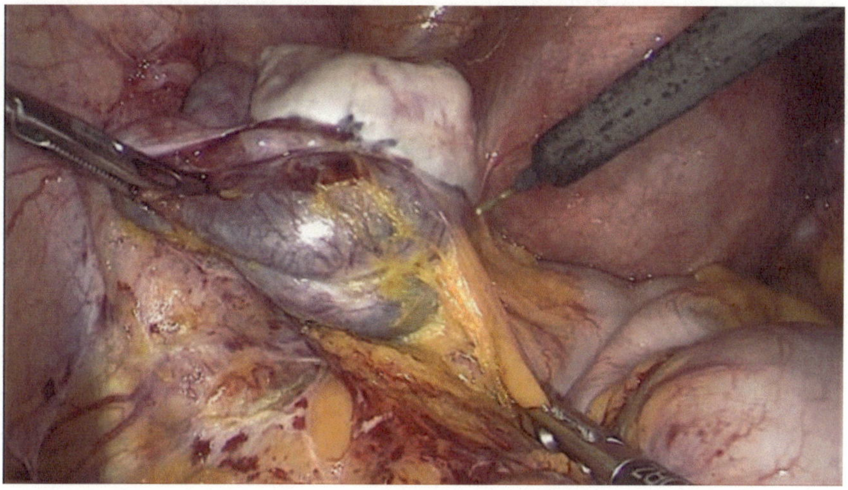

**Figure 5.** Excision of endometrioma using monopolar hook.

### 2.2.6. *Ovarian reserve*

As shown in this paper and in numerous studies, surgery performed on the ovaries may reduce the ovarian reserve and decrease the fertile potential in some women (especially infertile women with endometrioma or women with previous ovarian surgery) [4–8]. The ESHRE guideline for the management of women with endometriosis attempts to help these women and their physicians by suggesting surgical abstention, excepting cases of absolute indication [7].

In patients with disease-related symptoms, unilateral cysts, normal AMH, or sonographic features raising the suspicion for malignancy, ESHRE guidelines recommend surgery [8]. Another situation, where surgery is mandatory, is in patients who already have children. However, in all cases with endometriosis that are suitable for surgery, women should be counseled on the potential for decrease in ovarian reserve [14, 17].

Nevertheless, the decision for surgery in patients who are diagnosed with infertility should be taken with a lot of caution because several studies indicated that an endometrioma does not appear to adversely affect IVF outcomes and in the same time surgical excision of an endometrioma does not appear to improve IVF outcomes [15].

The most recent articles suggest that asymptomatic infertile patients, older patients, as well as those with diminished ovarian reserve or bilateral endometriomas, or those with prior surgical treatment, would benefit from proceeding directly to IVF [16].

Concerning the size of an endometrioma, it should be stressed that female patients with endometriomas less than 3 cm do not qualify for surgical treatment because the procedure of removing such a cyst decreases the ovarian reserve and does not positively influence the pregnancy rate. Small ovarian cysts less than 3 cm in diameter can be punctured and drained [7–10].

In 2012, the Practice Committee of the American Society for Reproductive Medicine no longer recommended performing laparoscopy on asymptomatic women with infertility to check for endometriosis [10–13].

More articles are reporting a reduction in ovarian reserve and antimulerrian hormone level after laparoscopic surgery for endometriomas. Frequently, during the surgery, normal ovarian tissue is excised with the endometrioma wall [10–14].

Ovarian surgery might reduce the number of oocytes retrieved, to reduce the peak estradiol levels and to increase total FSH requirement, in conclusion the fertility is very low reduced. It has been reported that ovarian surgery can lead to ovarian failure in 15% of the cases [20–22].

A study conducted by Donnez et al. showed that a combined technique of excisional (cystectomy) and laser ablative surgery without ovarian suture could be the best compromise for sparing ovarian reserve [4–7].

When revising the technique of laparoscopic cyst removal in regard of the ovarian reserve, many authors consider it more deleterious than the other technique of emptying the cyst and thermal coagulation or laser vaporization of its wall. The main argument is that during dissection and stripping of the cyst, the surgeon cannot completely avoid removal or damaging of the healthy ovarian parenchyma. In order to establish the superiority of one technique over the other, Tsolakidas et al. performed a comparative study between the laparoscopic cystectomy and a more conservative procedure consisting of a combination of three methods (drainage of the cyst and vaporization by laparoscopy followed by 3 months of GnRh analogue). The results showed that antimullerian hormone level does not decline in women who underwent the more conservative procedure compared to those who underwent the stripping procedure [18–20].

The idea of combining the two standardized procedures of cystectomy and of fenestration and vaporization was explored by Donnez et al. In his method, when approaching the hilus of the ovary, the excision of the cyst is stopped and $CO_2$ laser is applied on the remaining tissue. He managed to demonstrate that six months later the volume of the operated on ovary and AFC does not differ significantly from the opposite side [21, 22].

Therefore, the decision to proceed with surgery should be considered carefully if the patient had previous ovarian surgery or she does not have any child [18].

Further surgical procedures should not be attempted if initial surgery is not followed by a pregnancy, because it appears that fecundability is reduced or unaffected [23].

Moreover, it seems that the pregnancy rates decrease by almost twofolds in case of multiple procedures compared to initial surgery (22 vs. 40%) [23]. Indication for further surgical interventions must take into account several factors such as age, symptoms, ovarian reserve, the need for histological confirmation for certain type of cysts, and availability of skilled surgeons [20].

### *2.2.7. Deeply infiltrating endometriosis*

Usually, surgery for deeply infiltrating endometriosis is considered only if it is causing symptoms or if it might cause symptoms in the future. If surgical treatment is necessary, all the deep lesions must be excised in one operation to avoid the need for further surgery [19].

The therapy for symptomatic deeply infiltrating endometriosis is the resection with healthy margins. The operations often include partial rectum resection and partial resection of the sacrouterine ligament. Hysterectomy is not obligatory and is not wanted by the mostly young patients and a lot of doctors. The interventions can mostly be performed as laparoscopic and if necessary vaginal-assisted procedures (**Figure 6**) [20–23].

Concerning the deeply infiltrating endometriosis treatment, the 2012 National Institute for Health and Clinical Excellence (NICE) recommendations state that in case of conducting laparoscopy and finding possible stage-I or stage-II lesions, it is advisable to remove them, whereas for stage-III or stage-IV lesions, surgical treatment is the only method indicated [18–20].

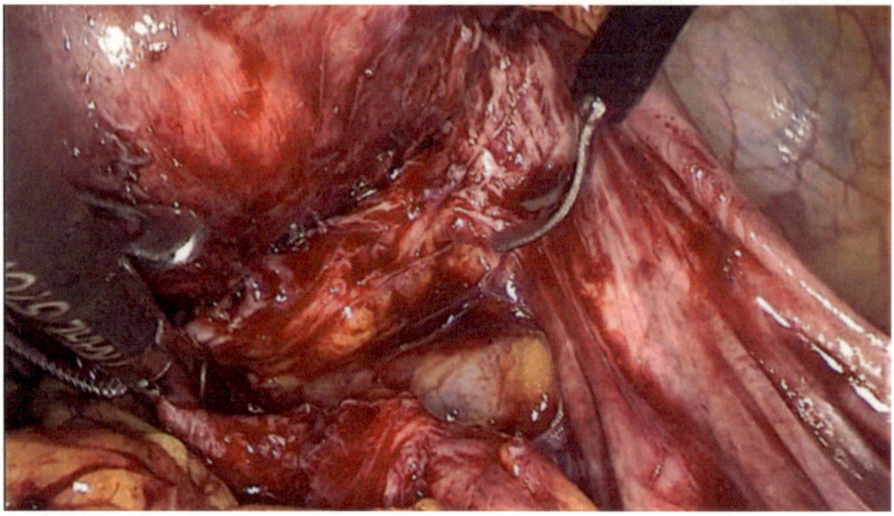

**Figure 6.** Dissection of deeply infiltrating endometriosis of the rectouterine pouch.

Auxiliary therapy after surgery is very important in order to eliminate or suppress residual lesions and prevent recurrence [21]. Advanced stage-III and stage-IV endometriosis will require surgical treatment consisting in the removal of the disease foci and restoring anatomical interrelations [22].

According to the American Society of Reproductive Medicine (ASRM), the treatment of stage-I and stage-II lesions with the use of laparoscopy slightly increases the percentage of pregnancies. In case of stage III and stage IV, correctly conducted laparoscopy significantly increases the percentage of pregnancies [18–23].

Laparoscopic uterine nerve ablation (LUNA) and laparoscopic presacral neurectomy (LPSN) are two procedures that involve cutting the nerves from the uterus in order to relieve chronic pain. Presacral neurectomy did provide better pain relief than laparoscopic treatment alone [10–12].

## 3. Conclusion

Pelvic endometriosis is a late diagnosed, complex, and in many aspects, a mysterious disease that still raises many questions and requires further research.

Nowadays, endometriosis can only be treated in up to 70% of cases with three major treatment options involving medical therapy, surgery, or combined treatment, with laparoscopy emerging as the main diagnostic and therapeutical tool for endometriosis and endometriomas. The most common surgical technique is stripping of the endometrioma; this technique can reduce ovarian reserve and decrease the chances of fertility.

There is controversial evidence regarding removal of endometriomas because of the potential impact on ovarian reserve, but there are also undisputable benefits of this type of surgery, such as pain relief.

Future research is needed to identify the optimal surgical techniques, as well as the prospects for new procedures such as aspiration with sclerotherapy or drainage with endometrial ablation by plasma laser energy, which may cause less ovarian damage while allowing the best clinical outcomes.

## 4. Disclosure

Sidonia Maria Saceanu, Stefan Patrascu, Anca Patrascu, Valeriu Surlin have nothing to disclose.

## Acknowledgements

Stefan Patrascu, Anca Patrascu, Valeriu Surlin have a contribution to the paper equal to that of the first author (Sidonia Maria Seceanu).

## Author details

Sidonia Maria Saceanu[1], Stefan Patrascu[2], Anca Patrascu[3] and Valeriu Surlin[2*]

*Address all correspondence to: vsurlin@gmail.com

1 Second Gynecology Department, University of Medicine and Pharmacy of Craiova, Craiova, Romania

2 First Clinic of Surgery, University of Medicine and Pharmacy of Craiova, Craiova, Romania

3 University of Medicine and Pharmacy of Craiova, Craiova, Romania

## References

[1] Ruan YQ, Liang WG, Huang SH. Analysis of laparoscopy on endometriosis patients with high expression of CA125. Eur Rev Med Pharmacol Sci. 2015;19:1334–1337. PMID: 25967705

[2] Burghaus S, Klingsiek P, Fasching PA, Engel A, Häberle L, Strissel PL, Schmidt M, Jonas K, Strehl JD, Hartmann A, Lermann J, Boosz A, Thiel FC, Müller A, Beckmann MW, Renner SP. Risk factors for endometriosis in a German case–control study. Geburtsh Frauenheilk. 2011;71:1073–1079. DOI: 10.1055/s-0031-1280436.

[3] Ke X, Qian H, Kang L, Wang J, Xie Y, Cheng Z. Clinical analyses of endometriosis after conservative surgery. Int J Clin Exp Med. 2015;8(11):21703–21706. PMID: 26885130

[4] Roustan A, Perrin J, Debals-Gonthier M, Paulmyer-Lacroix O, Agostini A, Courbiere B. Surgical diminished ovarian reserve after endometrioma cystectomy versus idiopathic DOR: comparison of in vitro fertilization outcome. Hum Reprod. 2015;30(4):840–847. DOI: 10.1093/humrep/dev029.

[5] Naufel DZ, Penachim TJ, de Freitas LL, Cardia PP, Prando A. Atypical retroperitoneal endometriosis and use of tamoxifen. Radiol Bras. 2014;47(5):323–325. DOI: 10.1590/0100-3984.2013.1774.

[6] De la Hera-Lazaro CM, Muñoz-González JL, Perez RO, Vellido-Cotelo R, Díez-Álvarez A, Muñoz-Hernando L, Alvarez-Conejo C, Jiménez-López JS. Radical surgery for endometriosis: analysis of quality of life and surgical procedure. Clin Med Insights Womens Health. 2016;9:7–11. DOI: 10.4137/CMWH.S38170.

[7] Younis A, Hawkins K, Mahini H, Butler W, Garelnabi M. Serum tumor necrosis factor-$\alpha$, interleukin-6, monocyte chemotactic protein-1 and paraoxonase-1 profiles in women with endometriosis, PCOS, or unexplained infertility. J Assist Reprod Genet. 2014;31: 1445–1451. DOI: 10.1007/s10815-014-0237-9.

[8] Fadhlaoui A, Bouquet de la Jolinière J, Feki A. Endometriosis and infertility: how and when to treat? Front Surg. 2014;1:24. DOI: 10.3389/fsurg.2014.00024.

[9] Jin X, Ruiz Beguerie J. Laparoscopic surgery for subfertility related to endometriosis: a meta-analysis. Taiwan J Obstet Gynecol. 2014;53(3):303–308. DOI: 10.1016/j.tjog.2013.02.004.

[10] Keyhan S, Hughes C, Price T, Muasher S. An update on surgical versus expectant management of ovarian endometriomas in infertile women. Biomed Res Int. 2015: 204792. DOI: 10.1155/2015/204792.

[11] Słabuszewska-Jóźwiak A, Ciebiera M, Baran A, Jakiel G. Effectiveness of laparoscopic surgeries in treating infertility related to endometriosis. Ann Agric Environ Med. 2015;22(2):329–331. DOI: 10.5604/12321966.1152089.

[12] Sanchez AM, Papaleo E, Corti L, Santambrogio P, Levi S, Viganò P, Candiani M, Panina-Bordignon P. Iron availability is increased in individual human ovarian follicles in close proximity to an endometrioma compared with distal ones. Hum Reprod. 2014;29(3): 577–583. DOI: 10.1093/humrep/det466.

[13] Dunselman GA, Vermeulen N, Becker C, Calhaz-Jorge C, D'Hooghe T, De Bie B, Heikinheimo O, Horne AW, Kiesel L, Nap A, Prentice A, Saridogan E, Soriano D, Nelen W; European Society of Human Reproduction and Embryology. ESHRE Guidelines:

management of women with endometriosis. Hum Reprod. 2014;29(3):400–412. DOI: 10.1093/humrep/det457.

[14] Kitajima M, Defrère S, Dolmans MM, Colette S, Squifflet J, Van Langendonckt A, Donnez J. Endometriomas as a possible cause of reduced ovarian reserve in women with endometriosis. Fertil Steril. 2011;96(3):685–691. DOI: 10.1016/j.fertnstert.2011.06.064.

[15] Chiang HJ, Lin PY, Huang FJ, Kung FT, Lin YJ, Sung PH, Lan KC. The impact of previous ovarian surgery on ovarian reserve in patients with endometriosis. BMC Womens Health. 2015;15:74. DOI: 10.1186/s12905-015-0230-1.

[16] Kitajima M, Dolmans M, Donnez O, Masuzaki H, Soares M, Donnez J. Enhanced follicular recruitment and atresia in cortex derived from ovaries with endometriomas. Fertil Steril. 2014;101(4):1031–1037. DOI: 10.1016/j.fertnstert.2013.12.049.

[17] Kuroda M, Kuroda K, Arakawa A, Fukumura Y, Kitade M, Kikuchi I, Kumakiri J, Matsuoka S, Brosens IA, Brosens JJ, Takeda S, Yao T. Histological assessment of impact of ovarian endometrioma and laparoscopic cystectomy on ovarian reserve. J Obstet Gynaecol Res. 2012;38(9):1187–1193. DOI: 10.1111/j.1447-0756.2012.01845.x.

[18] Qiu JJ, Liu YL, Liu MH, Chen LP, Xu DW, Zhang ZX, Yang QC, Liu HB. Ovarian interstitial blood flow changes assessed by transvaginal color Doppler sonography: predicting ovarian endometrioid cyst-induced injury to ovarian interstitial vessels. Arch Gynecol Obstet. 2012;285(2):427–433. DOI: 10.1007/s00404-011-1971-1.

[19] Barri PN, Coroleu B, Tur N, Barri-Soldevila PN, Rodrıguez I. Endometriosis-associated infertility: surgery and IVF, a comprehensive therapeutic approach. Reprod Biomed Online. 2010;21(2):179–185. DOI: 10.1016/j.rbmo.2010.04.026.

[20] Brosens I, Gordts S, Puttemans P, Benagiano G. Pathophysiology proposed as the basis for modern management of the ovarian endometrioma. Reprod Biomed Online. 2014; 28(2):232–238. DOI: 10.1016/j.rbmo.2013.09.024.

[21] Pearce CL, Templeman C, Rossing MA, Lee A, Near AM, Webb PM, Nagle CM, Doherty JA, Cushing-Haugen KL, Wicklund KG, Chang-Claude J, Hein R, Lurie G, Wilkens LR, Carney ME, Goodman MT, Moysich K, Kjaer SK, Hogdall E, Jensen A, Goode EL, Fridley BL, Larson MC, Schildkraut JM, Palmieri RT,Cramer DW, Terry KL, Vitonis AF, Titus LJ, Ziogas A, Brewster W, Anton-Culver H, Gentry-Maharaj A, Ramus SJ, Anderson AR, Brueggmann D, Fasching PA, Gayther SA, Huntsman DG, Menon U, Ness RB, Pike MC, Risch H, Wu AH, Berchuck A. Ovarian Cancer Association Consortium. Association between endometriosis and risk of histological subtypes of ovarian cancer: a pooled analysis of case-control studies. Lancet Oncol. 2012;13(4):385–394. DOI: 10.1016/S1470-2045(11)70404-1.

[22] Kim JY, Jee BC, Suh CS, Kim SH. Preoperative serum anti-mullerian hormone level in women with ovarian endometrioma and mature cystic teratoma. Yonsei Med J. 2013;54(4):921–926. DOI: 10.3349/ymj.2013.54.4.921.

[23] Dunselman GA, Vermeulen N, Becker C, Calhaz-Jorge C, D'Hooghe T, De Bie B, Heikinheimo O, Horne AW, Kiesel L, Nap A, Prentice A, Saridogan E, Soriano D, Nelen W. European Society of Human Reproduction and Embryology. ESHRE guideline: management of women with endometriosis. Hum Reprod. 2014;29(3):400–412. DOI: 10.1093/humrep/det457.

Chapter 4

# Laparoscopic Surgery in the Treatment of Endometriosis

Sonja Pop-Trajkovic Dinic, Jasmina Popovic,
Radomir Zivadinovic, Dejan Mitic,
Vladimir Antic and Milan Trenkic

Additional information is available at the end of the chapter

http://dx.doi.org/10.5772/65544

**Abstract**

Endometriosis is a benign disease, which affects about 10% of reproductive age women and almost 50% of infertile women. Although every year at least 300 new articles deal with this topic, endometriosis is still a enigmatic disease starting with theories of etiopathogenesis where there is still no consensus about the major cause of endometriosis. Also there is still no consensus about the management of the disease, mainly when there is an infertile patient who is preparing for *in vitro* fertilization procedure.

**Keywords:** disease, endometriosis, surgery, infertility, IVF

## 1. Introduction

Endometriosis is classically defined as the presence of endometrial glands and stroma in ectopic locations, primarily the pelvic peritoneum, ovaries, and rectovaginal septum. This benign disease affecting 6–10% of women of reproductive age, but the prevalence is as high as 35–50% if the women are infertile or experience chronic pelvic pain. Yet endometriosis is underdiagnosed and mean latency from onset of symptoms to definitive diagnosis is 6.7 years. Endometriosis is the third main indication for hysterectomy after endometrial carcinoma and different kind of bleeding connected to myomas [1, 2].

## 2. Etiopathogenesis of endometriosis

The major dilemma is always understanding the etiology and pathogenesis of this condition. The past several decades have witnessed substantial progress toward unraveling the enigma associated with this disorder [3].

### 2.1. Retrograde menstruation theory

The theory of retrograde menstruation is proposed by Sampson in the 1920s, both attractive and supported by multiple scientific evidences. According to this theory, eutopic endometrium is transferred through patent fallopian tubes into the peritoneal cavity during menstruation. The facts supporting this theory are next: The prevalence of endometriosis is high in adolescent girls with congenital obstructed or compromised tracts. Also in up to 90% of women with patent tubes undergoing laparoscopy during the perimenstrual time of the cycle, the menstrual blood is found in the pouch of Douglas. The larger volume of retrograde menstrual fluid found in the pelvises of patients with endometriosis when compared with healthy women may increase the risk of endometriotic lesion implantation. Escape from immune clearance, attachment to peritoneal epithelium, invasion of the epithelium, establishment of local neurovascularity, and continued growth and survival are necessary if endometriosis is to develop from retrograde passage of endometrium. However, this theory has been disputed in the past since it cannot explain the occurrence of endometriosis in pre-pubertal girls, newborns, or males [4–6].

### 2.2. Coelomic metaplasia theory

According to this theory, endometriosis originates from the metaplasia of cells, which are present in the mesothelial lining of the visceral and abdominal peritoneum. Transformation of normal peritoneal cells into endometrium-like cells is supported by hormonal or immunological background. This theory may explain the occurrence of disease in girls before puberty. However, main supporting factor, estrogen, is not present in the pre-pubertal girls and therefore this condition may be different from endometriosis that is found in women of reproductive age. Ectopic endometrial tissue has also been detected in female fetuses and therefore supported the theory of abnormal embryogenesis. This theory postulates that residual cells of the Wolffian or Mullerian ducts persist and develop into endometriotic lesions that respond to estrogen. Furthermore, recent theories suggest coelomic metaplasia to be the origin of adolescent variant of severe and progressive form of endometriosis. However, possible error of this theory is found in the fact that endometriotic lesions can also be found in areas outside of the course of Mullerian duct. It is stated by many studies that undifferentiated cells can differentiate into endometrial-like tissue. This process is induced by endogenous biochemical or immunological factors [7–10].

### 2.3. Stem cell theory

The existence of a stem cell pool is supported by the repetitive regeneration of the endometrium after menses and re-epithelialisation of the endometrium after any kind of artificial damage (curettage). The stem cells are supposed to exist in the basalis layer of the endometrium since the basalis layer of the endometrium is not shed with the monthly menstrual shedding of the functional layer. Recently, clonogenic cells have been identified and proposed to be involved in the formation of ectopic endometrial lesions. These cells are thought to represent the stem cell population in the human endometrium.

Stem cells are pluripotent cells. This means that they have ability to differentiate into one or several types of specialized cells. Differentiation is defined as a change in cell's gene expression, which leads to the alteration of the cell phenotype enabling the cell to have a specific function. The undifferentiated endometrial stem cells may be less responsive to ovarian steroids than the terminally differentiated cells due to lack of expression of hormone receptors. Retrograde menstruation can lead to the abnormal translocation of normal endometrial basalis, which can result in the involvement of stem cells in the formation of endometriotic deposits. Brosens et al. postulated that the uterine bleeding in neonatal girls contains a high amount of endometrial progenitor cells and that some of these cells may reside and reactivate in response to ovarian hormones later in life.

Leyendecker et al. proposed that women with endometriosis abnormally shed the endometrial basalis tissue, which, in combination with retrograde menstruation, initiates endometriotic deposits. The baboon model of endometriosis induction, where placement of the stem cell-rich endometrial basalis in the pelvic cavity resulting in 100% induction of endometriosis in all animals, may further support Leyendecker's theory.

Alternatively, these stem cells may be transported through the lymphatic or blood vessels to ectopic sites. The evidence that some of the endometrial stem cells have bone marrow origin further support the hematogenous dissemination theory of these cells. On the other hand, aberrant stem cell can relocate from the endometrium to an ectopic site and can generate endometrium-like lesions. Endometrial tissue produces several chemokines and angiogenic cytokines so this lesion can reside in the ectopic sites due to neovascularization.

The last possibility of stem cell involvement in endometriosis is the differentiation of the peritoneal, hematopoietic, or ovarian stem cells into endometrium-like tissue. Cytokines flow between uterine cavity and peritoneal cavity through the fallopian tubes. This connection may regulate the endometrium-like differentiation of resident stem cell population in the peritoneal cavity. Although possible, the reasons for such differentiation of the peritoneal stem cells into endometrium-like tissue in only up to 10% of the female population remain unexplained [11–21].

### 2.4. Inflammatory disease theory

There is a growing body of evidence that supports the concept of endometriosis as a pelvic inflammatory condition. In women with endometriosis, the peritoneal fluid is rich in activated macrophages and the cytokine/chemokine profile of it is different from the peritoneal fluid of women without endometriosis. In the peritoneal fluid of patients with endometriosis, one protein is identified, which is structurally similar to haptoglobin. This protein can bind to macrophages. That way it increases the production of IL-6 by macrophages and reduces their phagocytic activity. Some other cytokines, such as MIF (macrophage migration inhibitory factor), tumor necrosis factor (TNF)-a, interleukin (IL)-1b, and IL-6, can be found in the peritoneal fluid of women with endometriosis. Also chemoattractants such as IL-8, RANTES (Regulated on Activation, Normal T Cell Expressed and Secreted), and MCP-1/CCL2 (monocyte chemoattractant protein-1) can be identified in peritoneal fluid of the women with the disease. Yet, it is not clear if the observed cytokine profile is a cause or a consequence what remains to be definitively determined.

The peritoneal microenvironment in the setting of endometriosis is significantly richer in prostaglandins, and these mediators likely play a central role in the development of the disease as well as in its clinical presentation (pain and infertility). Peritoneal macrophages from women with endometriosis express higher levels of cyclo-oxygenase-2 (COX-2) and release significantly higher amounts of prostaglandins than macrophages from healthy women [22–24].

### 2.5. Hormonal disease theory

Hormonal alterations may influence the ability of endometrial cells to proliferate, attach to the mesothelium, and/or escape immune-mediated clearance. The concept of endometriosis as an estrogen-dependent disorder is well supported by molecular evidences. Crucial finding is that when we compare ectopic endometriotic tissue with eutopic increased activity of the aromatase enzyme and decreased activity of 17b-hydroxysteroid dehydrogenase (17b-HSD) type 2 is found. Increased aromatase activity is the consequence of the higher production of prostaglandin $E_2$ ($PGE_2$), which is stimulated by higher locally bioavailable $E_2$ concentration. These findings support the ability of endometriotic lesions for $E_2$ biosynthesis and confirm treatments, which supposed to lead to hypoestrogenism [25, 26].

### 2.6. Autoimmune disease theory

One very attractive theory claims that endometriosis occurs when defective immune response is present. This theory is supported by the fact that autoimmune diseases are found to be more common in women with endometriosis. Women with endometriosis have a higher concentration of activated macrophages, decreased cellular immunity, and a repressed NK cell function. Ectopic endometrial cells in the peritoneum induce an inflammatory response, and macrophages and leukocytes are activated locally. This inflammatory response may have negative influence which prevents elimination of ectopic endometrial cells that now can grow in ectopic sites [27–29].

### 2.7. Genetic disease theory

A genetic theory of endometriosis is supported by the familiar occurrence of the disease, by the existence of endometriosis in twins, and by the fact that women are in higher risk for the disease if their mothers were affected. A great number of studies have found that endometriosis has a polygenic mode of inheritance that is likely to involve multiple loci. Some chromosomal regions were reported to be associated with the corresponding endometriosis phenotype [30].

## 3. Symptoms of endometriosis

Symptoms of endometriosis primarily depend on its localization. The major symptoms are infertility, chronic pelvic pain, dysmenorrhea, and dyspareunia. Dyschezia appears predominantly in the cases when the endometriosis is localized on the rectovaginal septum, while bowel involvement leads to constipation, diarrhea, and meteorism. Dysuria and hematuria are present in the cases where endometriosis involves urinary bladder, as well as symptoms of ureteral obstruction with consequential hydronephrosis and deprivation of renal function on the side of involved ureter. In the rare cases, in which endometriosis involves pleura and lungs, hemoptysis, hemathorax, or pneumothorax may appear [31].

## 4. Diagnosis of endometriosis

Diagnosis of endometriosis is based on a specific symptomatology, clinical, and ultrasonographic presentation, but definitive confirmation is based on a videolaparoscopic visualization of the lesions and on a histological verification of endometrial glands and stroma. Combination of videolaparoscopy and histology is a "Golden standard" in the diagnosis of endometriosis. Sole laparoscopy can lead to a greater incidence of false positive diagnoses. From the other hand, endometriosis can be unrecognized if the laparoscopy is performed by an inexperienced surgeon.

Having the knowledge about the most frequent localization and the appearance of endometriosis is crucial in laparoscopic exploration. It is important, for the didactical reasons, to distinguish three morphological forms of the disease that can be seen throughout the laparoscopy: superficial endometriotic implants, endometriomas, and deep infiltrative endometriosis (DIE).

Diagnosis of the superficial peritoneal endometriosis is based on a laparoscopic evaluation with or without histological confirmation. Superficial peritoneal implants are most often localized on the uterosacral ligaments, in the pouch of Douglas, ovarian fossa, and on the lateral pelvic wall. In the rare cases, we can find them in the upper parts of the abdominal cavity, on the bladder surface, or on the surface of the intestines. For that reason, it is important to explore the whole abdominal cavity. The diagnosis of superficial peritoneal endometriosis is purely laparoscopic visualization with or without histological verification. Superficial peritoneal implants are usually localized to the uterosacral ligaments, Douglas string, ovarian fossa, and lateral pelvic walls. Less commonly, they can be found in the upper parts of the abdomen, on the surface of the bladder, and bowel. Therefore, we must make a full inspection of the abdomen. Superficial implants can be dark (brown and black) red and white. The dark lesion is found in moderate-to-severe stages of advanced endometriosis. Red lesions are presented as red hot fields, petechiae on the peritoneum, the fields of increased vascularization, and vesicular *ekrescence*: a sign of active endometriosis. Bright field in the form of white *scarified* lesions or very light brown boxes are signs of healed or latent endometriosis. Magnification received during laparoscopy allows visualization of very small lesions, 400–180 microns, and red to white lesions (**Figure 1**).

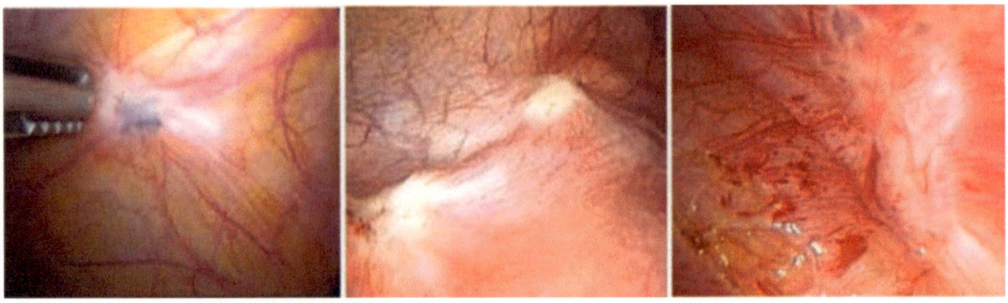

**Figure 1.** Superficial peritoneal endometriosis: dark, white and red lesions.

Diagnosis endometrioma is simple if they are over 2 cm and on the surface of the ovary (**Figure 2**). These endometriomas are detected on sonographic examination as opalescent hyperechogenic cystic changes whose descriptive echogenicity is compared with echogenicity of "the milky glass" (Ground-glass opacification—GGO—figure corresponded to pathomorphological substrate terr-chocolate cysts).However, small endometriomas can be found in as many as 48% of outside normal and enlarged ovaries. Preoperative ultrasound ovary examination is useful for the diagnosis of subcortical small endometrioma to be explored during the laparoscopy puncture.

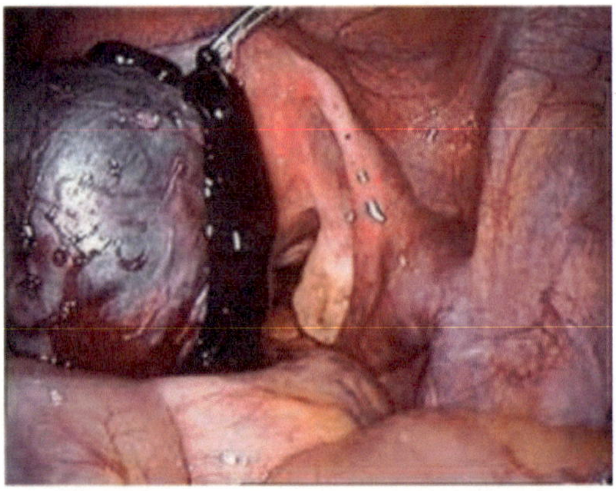

**Figure 2.** Endometrioma.

The deep infiltrative endometriosis (DIE) is defined by subperitoneal invasion of endometriotic lesions with a depth of penetration of more than 5 mm. It occurs to fibromuscular structures, primarily in the rectovaginal septum and *sacro uterine* connections (nearly 70%), vagina (14.5%), digestive system (about 10%), and urinary system (about 10%).The deep infiltrative endometriosis is an entity totally different from superficial endometriosis and endometrioma. A crucial argument in favor for this is the discovery that these lesions show no expression of HOX10 gene (associated with the endometrium), but 11 I 12 HOX genes (associated with the vagina and cervix), so it is considered that these nodules are actually the result of a tumor process, which originates from the cervix and the vagina. In less than 10% of cases, it can arise from metaplasia remains of Miller's channels [32]. The nodes of deep pelvic endometriosis can be clearly seen on MR images and endometriosis of rectovaginal septum at the transrectal sonographic examination. Endometriosis of rectovaginal septum and sacrouterine relations during the laparascopy should always be suspected in cases of obliteration of the Douglas pouch with dense adhesions and reports of "frozen pelvis" during laparoscopic exploration. However, given that these lesions are predominantly retroperitoneal, very often, they may remain unrecognized. Sometimes, just a small defect in the rectovaginal septum in the form of "peritoneal window" indicates a deep pelvic endometriosis (**Figure 3**).

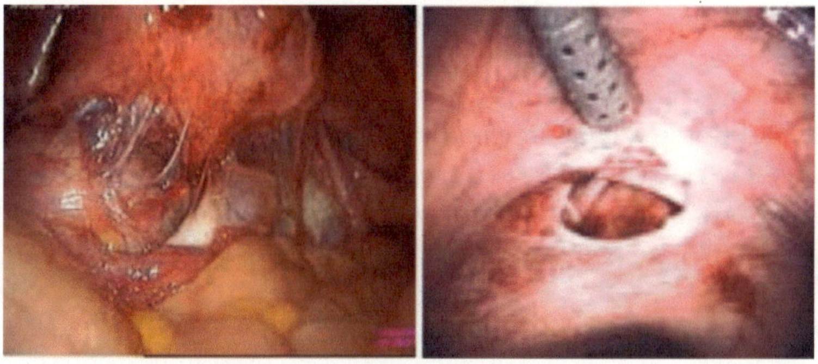

**Figure 3.** Deep infiltrative endometriosis: frozen pelvis and peritoneal window.

Diagnosis of endometriosis is missed in close to 7% as a lower stage in as many as 50% of cases. The classification is still mainly done by ASRM system (Revised American Society for Reproductive Medicine classification of endometriosis: 1996, 1997). Although there are many shortcomings, it is still used as the only internationally accepted classification. This classification was amended in 2005 with ENZIAN classification in terms of description and deep pelvic endometriosis and in 2010 EFI (Endometriosis Fertility Index) classification was released and it is applicable only to infertile patients [33]. A unique prognostic classification with clear guidelines still does not exist.

## 5. Surgery for endometriosis

Indications for video laparoscopic exploration are infertility, pain, or the presence of both symptoms. When planning the treatment, the following are taken into account: the patient's age, extent of the disease, the degree of severity of symptoms, and the desire to preserve fertility. The main guideline for the treatment is the need to preserve fertility. If this is the main symptom, the surgery is minimally extensive, especially when it comes to endometrioma. The main objective is not to reduce the ovarian reserve. If, on the other hand, the main symptom is the pain, the operation is maximum extensive in order to resolve the pain and prevent recurrence of the disease.

The first phase of the operation is to prepare the patient, the operating room, the team, and the equipment. This phase of work often determines the fate and success of the next stage in the surgical treatment and is as important as the possession of skills in endoscopic resolution of endometriosis. Patients with endometriosis require preoperative imaging processing that is necessary to clearly define the potential lesion preoperatively. "Bowel prep" or preparation for a potential digestive tract resection or segmental resection of the lesion of the "shaving" type is necessary in the case of anticipated ureteral endometriosis, and there is a possibility for preoperative placement of ureteral catheters or the same phase delay for a moment of resolving the ureteral endometriosis. Standard is a urethral catheterization. The patient is placed in dorsal litotomic gynecological position with the upper legs that are in the plane of the body with the mandatory setting of uterine manipulator (HUMI; Rumi, Valtchev, Koh, and others). Endoscopic team consists of gynecologist-operator, assistant, assistant to the manipulator, nurse, auxiliary nurse, nurses, and anesthesia team. We emphasize that the role of operators and assistants is almost equal in terms of responsibility for the success of surgery and that philosophy of endoscopic resolution of endometriosis is based on the assumption that the surgeon operator and assistants possess full doctrinal matching tie and technical approach to surgical treatment. The lesion is "attacked" by the operator and assistant with coordinated operation, using the safe techniques for dissection where the organization of a team and the mutual anticipation is a focal point in the work. Therefore, we recommend a team approach, i.e., engagement of previously cohesive teams with fully harmonized attitudes and knowledge to work. Since the surgery for endometriosis is one of the most complex, often more demanding than oncological endoscopic surgery, it is necessary to insist on the very thorough education of a surgeon who will determine endometriosis. The equipment consists of a trocar (umbilical —optical 5 or 10 mm depending on the telescope) and extra-ancelliar (two of 5 mm or three trocars out of which the third can be paraumbilically lateral or suprapubic), a telescope of 0 or 30 degrees, a system for suction and irrigation, bipolar forceps and scissors, dissecting and grasping forceps, laser system (optional), and harmonic system (optional).

After the introduction of optical and ancilliary trocar and creation of pneumoperitoneum, follows the detailed exploration of the pelvis and abdomen with a determination of the extension of the disease. Then follows the approach to adhesiolysis and the restoration of normal anatomic relationships. Adhesiolysis can be done by hydrosection, atraumatic forceps, bipolar or monopolar forceps, and scissors or Harmonic ultracision system (Ethicon US), depending on thickness and localization of adhesions.

Peritoneal implants may coagulate (by bipolar or unipolar currency), vaporize by using laser, or by excision. Any of these three techniques can be applied to lesions smaller than 2 mm. During the coagulation of the spots, we need to know that the depth of penetration can go from 20 mm for bipolar and even to 50 mm for monopolar energy. For lesions sized 3–5 mm laser vaporization or excision is used, while for those over 5 mm only excision is used. Prior to the excision, saline solution or Ringer lactate is injected retroperitoneally around the eye lesions (grasper is previously used to catch the lesion itself and transcend it to pick the peritoneum). This method of hydrodisection enables uplifting the peritoneal endometriotic implants from structures that may be below (ureter, blood vessels, and bladder). After this, an excision is performed around the implant of about 2 cm. This wide excision is suggested by the fact that one visible lesion of endometriosis is often accompanied by microscopic lesions around. The advantage of the excision technique is the possibility of histological verification of endometriosis.

Implants of endometriosis on the ovarian surface and endometriomas less than 2 cm can be coagulated, resected by laser, or excidated using scissors, bipolar, or accordion. These small endometriomas generally fall into type 1 endometrioma occurring by intussusception of superficial endometriosis implants, and it is very difficult to make excision on endometrioma capsules. When it comes to endometriomas larger than 3 cm, there are two surgical techniques: an ablative technique that involves drainage with aspiration of endometrioma content and then the destruction of the endometrioma wall by using laser or bipolar cautery. These techniques risk incomplete surgery and early endometrioma recurrence. Another technique involves the excision and "stripping" endometrioma capsules. Endometrioma excision begins with incision and aspiration of endometrioma content and then is repeatedly performed irrigation and aspiration of endometrioma cavity as well as inspection of the capsule walls (**Figure 4**). Incision is always done on the antimesenteric side of the ovary, as far as possible from the hilus. Then comes the dissecting plan or cleavage capsules to access the space between the capsule endometrioma and the ovarian tissue and then access the "stripping" of the capsule. This technique actually involves denudation of endometrioma using two grasping forceps that are used for traction and contractions. Applying these techniques means excessive risk of a surgery (removal of healthy ovarian tissue along with the capsule). The third technique combines the first two. Endometriomas larger than 3 cm generally fall into type 2 endometrioma occurring by infiltration of endometriosis in the corpus luteum. Depending on the depth of penetration of the implant, this technique can be simple and often complicated. In shallow penetration, endometrioma capsule can be fully removed. In deeper infiltration, insisting on complete removal of the capsule should not be the case. The existence of endometriosis in the ovary means that it threatens the healthy ovarian tissue and that the application of additional surgical techniques can significantly reduce the ovarian reserve. This is especially important for a group of infertile patients.

Although the original studies have indicated less damage to the ovary by applying ablative techniques, recent studies indicate increased rates of spontaneous conception to 2.5 times after excision techniques as well as to 4 times lower recurrence of chronic pelvic pain and 3 times lower risk of recurrence after this technique [34]. However, it has been proven that when removing the endometrioma capsule, in many cases, we have the healthy ovarian tissue with the capsule. Near the ovarian hilum, healthy ovarian tissue was found in 69% of cases, whereas away from the hilum in a small percentage only primordial follicles are found [35]. Therefore, if the "stripping" requires the application of force, it is necessary to apply a combination of excision and ablative techniques. The traction and contraction should be very carefully carried out as long as possible until the ovarian hilum is reached. Then, the process should be stopped, cut the capsule, and carefully coagulate the rest of endometrioma capsule. The point is not to approach to hilus too close where the bleeding can be caused and subsequent necessary coagulation can completely distort the vascularization of the ovary and consequently ovarian reserve. An alternative technique is called stripping, i.e., "inversion" in whose basis comes to the initial derivation of ovarian endometrioma, ovarium inversion through derivational ovarian incision, incision of endometrioma pseudocapsule on the site of its bottom, and finding the cleavage plan, whereby the denudation of the capsule is carried in the opposite direction from classic technique that goes from edges and moves to the bottom (**Figure 5**). This technique is promoted as a potentially more optimal approach to finding the correct avascular cleavage with minimal loss of ovarian tissue and minimal disruption of ovarian vascularization. After the excision of endometrioma, infertile patients not only have a greater chance of spontaneous conception but also a good outcome in the process of in vitro fertilization. The majority of studies indicate that the damage caused by the operation is rather quantitative than qualitative and that these patients in the process of in vitro fertilization require a larger amount in the ampoules stimulation and longer stimulation but they have the same rate of pregnancy and childbirth compared to patients with tubal infertility [36]. The operation of endometrioma recurrence is technically demanding and complicated. Except in cases of symptomatic endometriosis, it should be avoided, especially in infertile patients with recurrency to be involved in the process of artificial insemination. Patients two times operated from endometriosis have much less chance of spontaneous conception as well as significantly lower rate of pregnancy in in vitro fertilization procedure [37].

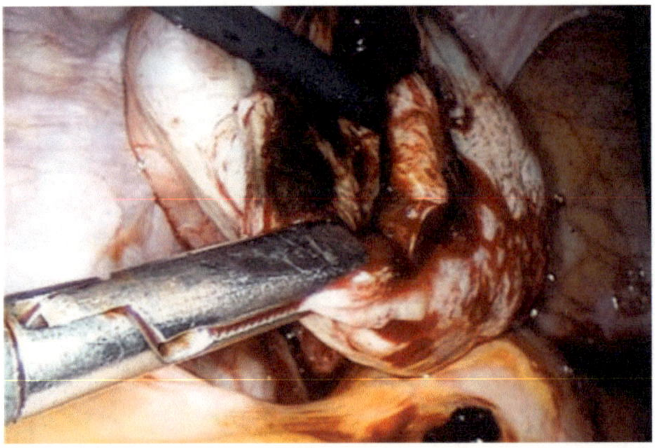

**Figure 4.** Incision and drainage of endometrioma.

In dealing with the DIE, the first postulate is the restoration of normal anatomic relationships in the pelvis. In order to have better access to the Douglas area, it is best to first empty the contents of endometrioma, release ovarian adhesions with the last leaf broad ligament, and temporarily fix them with a needle to the peritoneum of the anterior abdominal wall (System T-LIFT A. Wattiez-a is optimized for this maneuver). Maneuver of adnexal masses fixation is a "released hand" assistant who would otherwise be "trapped" by the need for the permanent removal of adnexal of the operative field. Then, we move on to identify the ureter. Given that

http://dx.doi.org/10.5772/65544

endometriosis is often a surgery of uterosacral ligaments and fibrosis medialises ureters, approach at this level is usually not safe. The simplest is to lift and incise the peritoneum at the level of "pelvic brim" (additus pelvis minoris-linea terminalis), laterally to the promontorium i a. iliacae communis and so access the ureter. Then, the downstream is followed and all the time it is lateralised. Laterally from a medial to the ureters, this internal iliac artery is the lateral aspect of pararectal fosse (Latzkov space), avascular space whose development ensures integrity of iliac vessels laterally, ureter medially and uterine arteries that is its front border and separating it from paravesicle fossa. The medial aspect of pararectal fossa is located medially to sacrouterine connections, and it is developed by peritoneal incision medial to sacrouterine relationship, sometimes even at the level of rectosigmoid and with blunt dissection, led by postulates that the fat belongs to the rectum, descend to the bottom of the medial aspect of pararectal fossa, the level of levatory panels and clearly show rectovaginal septum, rectum and vagina stub and define a proximal point of rectovaginal cleavage from which the rectal dissection is started as well as the separation from the rectum Denonvilliers's fascia at the level where the nodule DIE is present. Excision of endometriosis in this segment can be relatively simple, without compromising the integrity of the wall of the rectum or vagina. In the space of pararectal fossa, the position of the hypogastric nerve should be respected, and it is mostly freely compared to endometrioid lesions that in rare cases is affected by the disease when impossible to avoid his sacrifice. If the nodule affects vaginal mucosa or penetrates below the lamina muscularis mucosae rectum, then the rectal wall discoid resection or segmental resection of the rectum is performed, with or without resection of the vagina affected by the disease. "Rectal shaving" is a surgical principle applicable when a nodule of endometriosis rectum is superficial and does not penetrate to the mucosa. It implies "shaving" of rectal serosa with scissors along with meticulous and nonpenetrative hemostasis and with optional *reseroziranje* of the part of the rectum, which is exempt from endometriosis. Discoid resection of rectal wall involves removing the entire wall of the rectum, which is affected by the disease but not the entire sigmoid segment. Optimal embodiment is the use of circular staplers. Segmental resection of the rectum requires good mezorectal dissection and preparation for the placement of a circular stapler, which realizes the resection and T-T anastomoses at the same time.

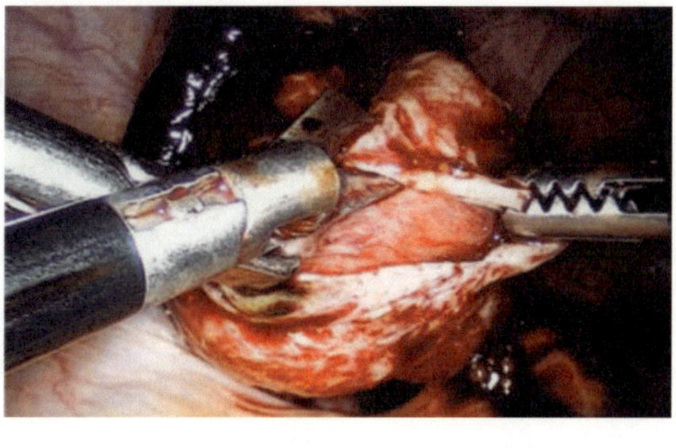

**Figure 5.** Stripping technique.

Ureteral endometriosis is manifested by hydroureter above the place of compression or obstruction node infiltration into the ureter with possible consequent hydronephrosis to a complete loss of kidney function on the affected side. The surgical approach involves a clear definition of the earlier mentioned positions of the ureter and its way through a small pelvis, developing pararectal and paravesicle fossa in order to clearly define the relationship of the ureter and blood vessels, and their preservation, and defining the degree and length of lesion. Compressive fibro-endometriotic "muff," which only compresses the urethra without destruction of the wall, is removed by precise and blunt dissection with the preservation of adventitial blood vessels of the ureter. When there is a "crush" lesion of the ureter or partial involvement of lumen in endometriosis nodule, the proximal and distal ureteral mobilization with ureteral resection is done, as well as the placement pig-tail ureteral (double J) catheter with termino-terminal anastomosis.

Endometriosis of the bladder may require the resection only of the part of serosa (superficial lesions), or if the nodule is transmural with mucosa affection, the resection of the bladder wall is done along with a suture in one or two or sometimes three layers with a mandatory catheterization next 2 weeks.

Treatment of deep pelvic endometriosis primarily aims to solve the pain. Regarding spontaneous conception after solving DIE, data from the literature are different, and the percentages range from 24% to 36% [38]. The impact of the success of solving DIE on VTO procedures that follow is still unclear.

Therefore, if an operation is performed on infertile patients, the treatment of endometriosis includes adhesiolysis, excision and coagulation of superficial endometriosis implants, stripping of endometrioma, and resolving of deep infiltrative endometriosis especially when infertility is associated with pain. When it comes to addressing chronic pelvic pain in patients who have completed the reproduction and do not want to preserve fertility, radical treatment should be taken into consideration. Extension of the disease does not affect much the intensity of the pain so that the removal of adhesions and endometriosis spots will, in some women, resolve the problem, especially if a deep pelvic endometriosis is solved, whereas the others require adnexectomy or hysterectomy. One optional technique is presacral neurectomy. This technique involves access to hypogastric plexus at the level of promontorium and removal of all fibers in interiliac triangle.

Given the fact that the endoscopic surgery for endometriosis is one of the most challenging and the most invasive in terms of the manipulation of tissues and organs of the pelvis, and that in the process of the excision of the disease, very vulnerable structures (iliac vessels, uterine blood vessels, ureters, bladder and bowel) are often approached, the percentage of complications (intra or perioperative) is greater than in the treatment of other benign conditions.

Blood vessel injuries occur most commonly during the excision of endometriosis from the lateral compartment during adhesiolysis and ovarium deliberation, which are captured in ovarian fossae or during the deliberation of the ureter. The most common reason is the inadequate implementation of energy or force of traction on the wall of the blood vessel or adhesiolysis method (sharp precise dissection or large force of blunt dissection). Injuries could be resolved with a ligature of blood vessels (if they are not vital and whose "sacrifice" does not jeopardize the function) or with wall suture (iliac blood vessels, aorta, and vena cava). Complications are endoscopically solvable as well, if the team that solves them is familiar with the endoscopic method of treatment.

Intestine injuries (usually rectosigmoid segment or the small intestine) occur during adhesiolysis or inadequate application of energy or the wrong assessment of the initial approach to solve endometrioid nodes (selection of rectal shaving in case the disease spread to the entire wall of the rectum and when it is necessary to open the intestinal lumen). Intraoperative complications are primarily unrecognized lesions of the intestinal wall and rectovaginal fistula or intestinal obstruction is postoperative.

Urinary complications are the result of removing the disease from the wall of the bladder or ureter complications but they are considered complications only in the case of same result of inadequate implementation of operational strategy in relation to the real state of the disease (segmental resection of the ureter with the ureteral endometriosis is not considered a complication but a planned surgical treatment, while ureteral resection because of the incidental ureteral injuries due to an inadequate use of force or energy is a complication).

Loss of ovarian reserves and POF is considered a very significant complication of fertility-preserving operative treatment, and in this sense there is a consensus that provides for the abandonment of excision surgery at the ovarium level on endometrioma less than 2 cm or those that affect almost the entire volume of the ovary or ovarian hilus and in patients with preoperative low ovarian reserve (estimated levels of AMH, AFC). Then, the derivative of endometrioma with partial destruction of zones of endometriosis in pseudocapsule is a surgical method of choice. In other cases, it is decided on the stripping of the capsule with all the above principles to achieve preservation of ovarian vascularization and residual ovarian function.

In order to prevent "seeding" or implantation of endometrioid tissue in the anterior abdominal wall at the site of trocar-incision, as one of the possible complications, it is an imperative to use a ENDOBAG when extracting the material at the end of the operation (pseudocapsule of endometrioma, implants, and nodules). Extraction way is usually on the side or umbilical incision on the skin [39].

## Author details

Sonja Pop-Trajkovic Dinic[1*], Jasmina Popovic[1], Radomir Zivadinovic[2], Dejan Mitic[2], Vladimir Antic[1] and Milan Trenkic[1]

*Address all correspondence to: sonjapoptrajkovic@gmail.com

1 Clinic for Gynecology Obstetrics, Nis, Serbia

2 Medical Faculty University of Nis, Clinic for Gynecology and Obstetrics Clinical Center of Nis, Nis, Serbia

## References

[1] L. C. Giudice. Endometriosis. The New England Journal of Medicine. 2010; 362(25): 2389–2398

[2] M. M. Carneiro, I. D. D. S. Filogônio, L. M. P. Costa, I. De Ávila, and M. C. Ferreira, Accuracy of clinical signs and symptoms in the diagnosis of endometriosis. Journal of Endometriosis. 2010; 2(2):63–70

[3] R. O. Burney and L. Giudice. Pathogenesis and pathophysiology of endometriosis. Fertility and Sterility. 2012;98(3):511–519

[4] P. R. Koninckx, D. Barlow, and S. Kennedy. Implantation versus infiltration: the Sampson versus the endometriotic disease theory. Gynecologic and Obstetric Investigation. 1999; 47(1):3–10

[5] P. R. Koninckx, A. Ussia, L. Adamyan, A. Wattiez, and J. Donnez. Deep endometriosis: definition, diagnosis, and treatment. Fertility and Sterility. 2012; 98(7):564–571

[6] J. A. Sampson. Heterotopic or misplaced endometrial tissue. American Journal of Obstetrics and Gynecology. 1925; 10(5):649–664

[7] A. Valentijn, H. Al-Lamee, K. Palial, et al. SSEA-1 Isolates human endometrial basal glandular epithelial cells: phenotypic and functional characterisation and implications in pathogenesis of endometriosis. Human Reproduction. 2013; 28(4): 2695–2708

[8] W. P. Dmowski and E. Radwanska. Current concepts on pathology, histogenesis and etiology of endometriosis. Acta Obstetricia et Gynecologica Scandinavica. 1984; 63(123):29–33.

[9] I. Brosens and G. Benagiano. Is neonatal uterine bleeding involved in the pathogenesis of endometriosis as a source of stem cells. Fertility and Sterility. 2013; 100(22):622–623

[10] P. Gruenwald. Origin of endometriosis from the mesenchyme of the celomic walls. American Journal of Obstetrics and Gynecology. 1942; 44(3):470–474

[11] H. M. Albertsen, R. Chettier, P. Farrington, and K. Ward. Genome-wide association study link novel loci to endometriosis. PLoS One. 2013; 8: Article ID e5825, 22–25.

[12] K. E. May, J. Villar, S. Kirtley, S. H. Kennedy, and C. M. Becker. Endometrial alterations in endometriosis: a systematic review of putative biomarkers. Human Reproduction Update. 2011; 17(5):637–653

[13] Y. Afshar, J. Hastings, D. Roqueiro, J. W. Jeong, L. C. Giudice, and A. T. Fazlebas. Changes in eutopic endometrial gene expression during the progression of experimental endometriosis in the baboon, *Papio anubis*. Biology of Reproduction. 2013; 88(3):44

[14] M. A. Khan, J. Sengupta, S. Mittal, and D. Ghosh. Genome-wide expressions in autologous eutopic and ectopic endometrium of fertile women with endometriosis. Reproductive Biology and Endocrinology. 2012; 10(8):84

[15] S. Tsuji, M. Yoshimoto, K. Takahashi, Y. Noda, T. Nakahata, and T. Heike. Side population cells contribute to the genesis of human endometrium. Fertility and Sterility. 2008;90(4):1528–1537

[16] H. A. Padykula. Regeneration in the primate uterus: the role of stem cells. Annals of the New York Academy of Sciences. 1991; 622:47-56.

[17] J. A. Deane, R. C. Gualano, and C. E. Gargett. Regenerating endometrium from stem/progenitor cells; is it abnormal in endometriosis, Asherman's syndrome and infertility? Current Opinion in Obstetrics and Gynecology. 2013; 25:193–200

[18] K. Kato. Stem cells in human normal endometrium and endometrial cancer cells: characterization of side population cells. Kaohsiung Journal of Medical Sciences. 2012;28(2):63-71

[19] F. R. Oliveira, C. D. Cruz, H. L. del Puerto, Q. T. M. F. Vilamil, F. M. Reis, and A. F. Camargos. Stem cells: are they the answer to the puzzling etiology of endometriosis? Histology and Histopathology. 2012;27(1):23–29

[20] C. E. Gargett, R. W. S. Chan, and K. E. Schwab. Hormone and growth factor signaling in endometrial renewal: role of stem/progenitor cells. Molecular and Cellular Endocrinology. 2008;288(1-2):22-29

[21] H. S. Taylor. Endometrial cells derived from donor stem cells in bone marrow transplant recipients. Journal of the American Medical Association. 2004;292(1):81-85

[22] H. Masuda, Y. Matsuzaki, E. Hiratsu et al. Stem cell-like properties of the endometrial side population: implication in endometrial regeneration. PLoS One. 2010;5(4): Article ID e10387, 121–123

[23] S. Gupta, A. Agarwal, N. Krajcir, and J. G. Alvarez. Role of oxidative stress in endometriosis. Reproductive BioMedicine Online. 2006;13(1):126-134

[24] A. Augoulea, A. Alexandrou, M. Creatsa, N. Vrachnis, and I. Lambrinoudaki. Pathogenesis of endometriosis: the role of genetics, inflammation and oxidative stress. Archives of Gynecology and Obstetrics. 2012; 5(1):1–5

[25] C. Parente Barbosa, A. M. Bentes De Souza, B. Bianco, and D. M. Christofolini. The effect of hormones on endometriosis development. Minerva Ginecologica. 2011;63(4): 375–386

[26] J. J. Kim, T. Kurita, and S. E. Bulun. Progesterone action in endometrial cancer, endometriosis, uterine fibroids, and breast cancer. Endocrine Reviews. 2013;34(2):130-162

[27] N. Sinaii, S. D. Cleary, M. L. Ballweg, L. K. Nieman, and P. Stratton. High rates of autoimmune and endocrine disorders, fibromyalgia, chronic fatigue syndrome and

atopic diseases among women with endometriosis: a survey analysis. Human Reproduction. 2002;17(10):2715–2724

[28] J. Sikora, A. Mielczarek-Palacz, and Z. Kondera-Anasz. Role of natural killer cell activity in the pathogenesis of endometriosis. Current Medicinal Chemistry. 2011;18(2):200-208.

[29] Y. Osuga, K. Koga, Y. Hirota, T. Hirata, O. Yoshino, and Y. Taketani. Lymphocytes in endometriosis. American Journal of Reproductive Immunology. 2011;65(1):1-10

[30] H. M. Albertsen, R. Chettier, P. Farrington, and K. Ward. Genome-wide association study link novel loci to endometriosis. PLoS One. 2013;8:Article ID e58257

[31] Bellelis P, Dias JA, Jr., Podgaec S, Gonzales M, Baracat EC and Abrão MS. Epidemiological and clinical aspects of pelvic endometriosis—a case series. Revista de Associacao Medica Brasileira 2010;56:467–471.

[32] Kulp, J. L., Cakmak, H. and Taylor, H. S. HOX Genes and Endometriosis, in Endometriosis: Science and Practice (eds L. C. Giudice, J. L. H. Evers and D. L. Healy), 2011. Wiley-Blackwell, Oxford, UK.

[33] Adamson GD. Endometriosis Fertility Index: is it better than the present staging systems? Current Opinion in Obstetrics & Gynecology. 2013; 25(3):186–92.

[34] Hart RJ, Hickey M, Maouris P, Buckett W. Excisional surgery versus ablative surgery for ovarian endometriomata. Cochrane Database Systematic Review 2008; 2: CD004992.

[35] Muzii L, Panici PB. Combined technique of excision and ablation for the surgical treatment of ovarian endometriomas: the way forward? Reproduction Biomedicine Online. 2010;20(2):300–2.

[36] Ruiz-Flores FJ and Garcia-Velascoa JA. Is there a benefit for surgery in endometrioma associated infertility? Current Opinion in Obstetrics & Gynecology 2012;24(3):136–140

[37] Berlanda D, Vercellini P and Fedele L. The outcome of repeat surgery for recurrent symptomatic endometriosis. Current Opinion in Obstetrics & Gynecology 2010; 22(4): 320–325

[38] Kondo W, Bourdel N, Tamburro S, Cavoli D, Jardon K, Rabischong B, Botchorishvili R, Pouly J, Mage G, Canis M. Complications after surgery for deeply infiltrating pelvic endometriosis. BJOG 2011; 118(3):292–8.

[39] deZiegler D, Borghese B, Chapron C. Endometriosis and infertility: pathophysiology and management. Lancet 2010;376(9742):730–8.

Chapter 5

# Deep Neuromuscular Blockade Improves Surgical Conditions During Gynecological Laparoscopy

Christophe Dransart, Laurie Putz,
Maria-Laura Marotta and Philippe E. Dubois

Additional information is available at the end of the chapter

http://dx.doi.org/10.5772/64934

**Abstract**

Obtaining an appropriate laparoscopic workspace depends on several factors related to the patient (i.e., weight and abdominal compliance) and the procedure (i.e., body's position, depth of anesthesia and intra-abdominal (IA) pressure). Among them, a deep neuromuscular blockade (NMB) contributes to provide the surgeon with better operating conditions. This chapter discusses the interests and challenges of muscle relaxation during gynecological laparoscopy. The introduction of sugammadex into clinical practice provides the opportunity to modify the management of neuromuscular blockade to improve the surgical conditions during laparoscopy as well as the safety of the patients. The maintenance of a rocuronium-induced deep neuromuscular block from the trocar insertion until the end of laparoscopy is no longer incompatible with rapid recovery and awakening in optimal conditions. Neuromuscular transmission (NMT) monitoring is the key to adequate management and should be used in all cases. Objective measurements allow for excellent intubation and surgical conditions, the definition of thresholds and doses for the administration of reversal agents, and the exclusion of residual blockade prior to the patient extubation.

**Keywords:** neuromuscular blockade, laparoscopic surgical conditions, rocuronium, neostigmine, sugammadex

## 1. Introduction

Since the first laparoscopy was performed on a human by Jacobaeus in Sweden in 1910 [1], laparoscopic techniques have steadily developed. It was not until 1943 that the first diagnostic gynecological laparoscopy was performed with uterine mobilization, thanks to Raoul Palmer's ingenuity [2]. In the 1950s, with the advent of a safer laparoscopic lighting system, laparoscopy had taken a step forward but remained mostly a diagnostic tool [3]. In 1982, the addition of a video camera to laparoscopes allowed surgeons to be helped by assistants and to perform more and more surgical techniques by laparoscopy (e.g., adhesiolysis, appendectomy, cholecystectomy, and hysterectomy) [2, 3].

Diagnostic laparoscopy became part of fertility work-ups, with the growing development of assisted reproductive technology (intrauterine inseminations and *in vitro* fertilization). When cost-effectiveness debates began, routine diagnostic laparoscopy was increasingly supplanted by these treatments. Nevertheless, surgical laparoscopy to treat advanced-stage endometriosis, tubal pathology, and ovarian cysts or to perform myomectomy remains beneficial [4–7].

Relative limitations of performing surgical laparoscopy are surgeon expertise (in fertility surgery), general anesthesia, patient obesity, cardiovascular disease (less frequent in young patients receiving fertility treatments), and previous abdominal surgery [3–5].

In the last few years, new techniques emerged providing the surgeon with high precision and less invasive tools (robotically assisted laparoscopy, single-port laparoscopy) [3, 8–11]. However, all laparoscopic procedures need to create a space inside the abdomen: the pneumoperitoneum.

## 2. The laparoscopic workspace

When insufflating the intra-abdominal (IA) cavity with gas, numerous elements contribute to provide the surgeon with an adequate space to work. Some depend on the patient and others on the procedure (**Figure 1**).

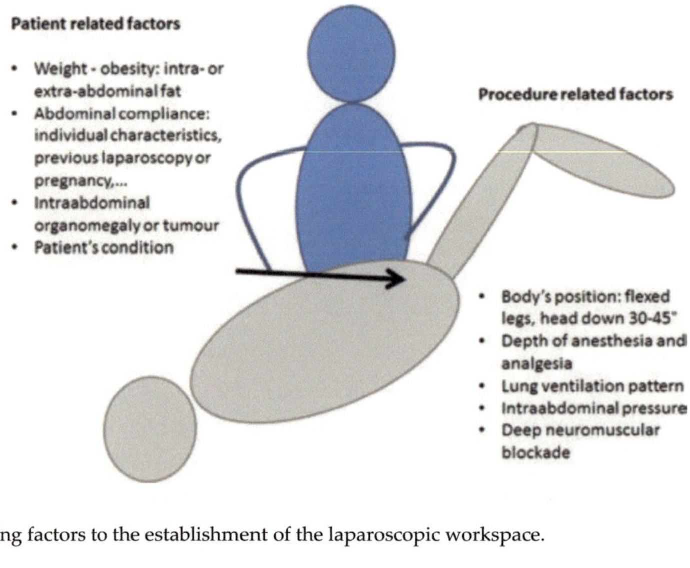


**Figure 1.** Contributing factors to the establishment of the laparoscopic workspace.

### 2.1. Weight

When creating the laparoscopic workspace in overweight or obese patients, difficulties are encountered due to the placement of laparoscopic trocars, with a higher risk of bleeding from abdominal wall vessels due to a restricted operative field limited by the thick abdominal wall or IA fat, and also due to limitations in placing obese patients in the Trendelenburg position [3]. To decrease the risk of bowel injury during under-umbilical laparoscopic entry, different techniques can be used: open under-umbilical laparoscopy or left/right upper-quadrant trocar insertion [3, 12].

### 2.2. Previous abdominal surgery

Fibrosis and adhesions can be barriers to the creation of a large IA workspace.

### 2.3. Previous pregnancy or laparoscopy

On the contrary, a previous muscular stretching of the abdominal wall could have modified the abdominal compliance in favor of larger IA volume [13].

### 2.4. Patient's anatomy

Any IA tumor or organomegaly can constitute a threat for laparoscopic entry and adequate workspace. In the case of huge or multiple fibroids (>10 cm in size), laparoscopic myomectomy cannot be performed, and laparotomy is then indicated [12].

### 2.5. Depth of anesthesia and analgesia

Anesthesiologists are obligated to provide the patient with safe care during surgery. This includes an adequate level of anesthesia and analgesia, considering the procedure requirements and the patient's health status. The anesthesiologist must, in collaboration with the surgeon, find the balance between benefits and harm of applying deep anesthesia during laparoscopy to improve the quality of surgical conditions. Their common goal is to perform safe and fast surgery under the best obtainable conditions.

### 2.6. The patient's body position

The body position significantly influences the abdominal inflation volume and, thus, could improve or worsen the surgical workspace. The mean inflated volume can be increased up to 900 mL in the Trendelenburg position and/or when the legs are slightly flexed at the hips [13, 14].

### 2.7. Intra-abdominal pressure (IAP)

Insufflating gas in the abdominal cavity during laparoscopy allows the creation of a workspace between the abdominal wall and the IA organs, the pneumoperitoneum.

The measurement of abdominal compliance makes it possible to estimate the required pressure needed to achieve a certain IA volume and explain why certain patients have a limited abdominal workspace compared with others during laparoscopy. The abdominal pressure-inflated volume relationship behaves in a linear fashion between 0 and 12 mmHg. Every abdomen can be described by two parameters: elastance and the pressure at zero volume [15].

In clinical practice, IAP is routinely monitored at 12–15 mmHg [16]. Low IAP is defined as 6–10 mmHg [17]. Low IAP has potential benefits when compared with standard pressure:

- Fewer adverse effects on pulmonary function [18]. However, blood gas analyses and pulmonary function tests are not significantly different. Healthy individuals, with the aid of artificial ventilator adjustments, are able to compensate for pulmonary function reduction during pneumoperitoneum [17]. Further studies are necessary for ASA three to four patients.

- Fewer hemodynamic side effects are encountered, including reduced preload and decreased cardiac output [19], but this does not seem to have significant advantages when compared with standard IAP in healthy patients [17].

- No significant or persistent liver (transient elevation of liver enzymes such as AST and ALT) or renal impairment (reduced renal perfusion, decreased urine output, but no changes in postoperative creatinine) was observed or had clinical consequences in healthy patients [17].

- Postoperative peritoneal adhesions and anastomotic leakage are important complications following gynecological and abdominal surgery. The mechanism is unclear but could include local hypoxemia caused by mechanical compression of the capillary bed reducing blood flow. Local hypercapnia induces acidosis and an impaired microcirculation [17]. One human study suggests that low IAP minimizes the adverse effects on surgical peritoneal environment [20].

- As with the head-down position, elevated IAP increases intrathoracic pressure, reduces cerebral venous drainage, and increases cerebrospinal fluid and subsequently intracranial and intraocular pressure [17].

- Low IAP is associated with significantly lower postoperative inflammatory response of IL2, IL6, and CRP [17, 21]. This has to be confirmed by further studies.

- Low IAP was associated with less postoperative pain during the early postoperative phase [22–24], including less shoulder referred pain [25–27]. This was also demonstrated after laparoscopic gynecologic procedures [28, 29]. Extended wash out of IA gas (5 min with open valve umbilical trocar after lap hysterectomy) was found to be an effective and safe method of reducing postoperative abdominal and shoulder pain levels [30].

A clinically significant reduction in pain score is likely to result in shorter hospital stays and earlier return to normal activity and work [31]. However, the difference in pain intensity between low and standard IAP was not always immediately significant, only after 2–3 days [17]. In addition, the reduction in postoperative analgesic requirement was not always relevant [22, 32]. Factors implicated in pain after laparoscopic surgery include diaphragm and phrenic nerve irritation or stretching, intraperitoneal acidosis, residual IA gas, volume and lack of humidity of the insufflated gas, wound size and the presence of drains, and also sociocultural and individual factors [31, 33, 34].

On the other hand, low IAP was often associated with a substantial reduction in visibility and available working space [35]. Then, decreasing IA pressure might prolong operation time and subsequently increase the costs of the procedure; this was not found to be significant [36]. Low pressure apparently resulted in a less than optimal surgical field, which could result in an increased incidence of surgical complications. However, low IAP had a comparable incidence of serious adverse events and conversions to open procedures when compared with standard pressure [28, 37, 38].

Finally, recommendations to use low IAP are weak, and more studies are required to establish the safety of low-pressure pneumoperitoneum and to explore its value for physicians and patients [17]. A practical and reasonable approach is to start with the lowest possible IAP that is required to obtain adequate exposure of the operative field [39] and to increase the pressure to routine level when the exposure is inadequate [40].

### 2.8. Is there a place for deep neuromuscular blockade (NMB) to improve the laparoscopic workspace and surgical conditions?

Neuromuscular blocking agents (NMBAs) were introduced into clinical practice in 1942 and were rapidly adopted as an important part of modern balanced anesthesia [41]. At a time when anesthesia was tricky in most patients, inducing a NMB significantly improved surgical conditions in more and more situations [42]. However, almost as soon as its use began, NMBA administration was associated with side effects and related mortality [43].

To secure the airway, orotracheal intubation is traditionally performed after injecting a NMBA. Compared with other techniques, excellent intubating conditions are more easily obtained with NMB and are less frequently associated with postoperative hoarseness and vocal cord injuries [44].

Classically, administering NMBA continuously during some surgical procedures may enhance patient safety and decrease morbidity (e.g., open eye surgery under general anesthesia and intracranial surgery) [31], but new indications emerged with the development of surgery, including laparoscopy [45]. The major determinant of the amount of pressure that is required for adequate surgical conditions is the compliance of the abdominal wall, which could be increased significantly by the administration of NMBA [17]. Madsen and colleagues also suggest that the possible negative effects of low-pressure pneumoperitoneum on perioperative conditions might be overcome by the adequate use of NMBA [46].

The goal of this chapter is to provide the reader with the factors that help to determine the benefits and challenges of maintaining a deep NMB during pelvic laparoscopy to improve the surgical workspace and the operating conditions.

## 3. Neuromuscular transmission: physiology and monitoring

The neuromuscular junction is the chemical step that transduces the electrical activity of a motor nerve ending to the postjunctional muscle membrane to ultimately generate muscle contraction (**Figure 2a**). The presynaptic nerve ending is responsible for acetylcholine (ACh) synthesis, packaging into vesicles, and release when the nerve membrane depolarizes. The synaptic cleft allows for rapid diffusion of the neurotransmitter. The postsynaptic membrane is a specialized region of folded muscle membrane filled with nicotinic acetylcholine receptors. Two acetylcholine molecules have to fix on the nicotinic receptor to open its ionic channel and, when numerous enough, induce the muscle membrane depolarization and the propagation of the electric signal, which generate the muscle contraction. ACh is rapidly inactivated and divided into acetate and choline by acetylcholinesterases present in the postsynaptic membrane folds. A presynaptic mechanism allows for sustained transmitter release over time to maintain the muscle contraction. When stimulated by ACh, slightly different nicotinic receptors present on the presynaptic nerve terminal mobilize storage vesicles to reach the nerve membrane and release a higher quantity of ACh in the synaptic cleft. This positive feedback mechanism allows for high intensity and long-duration muscle contraction [47].

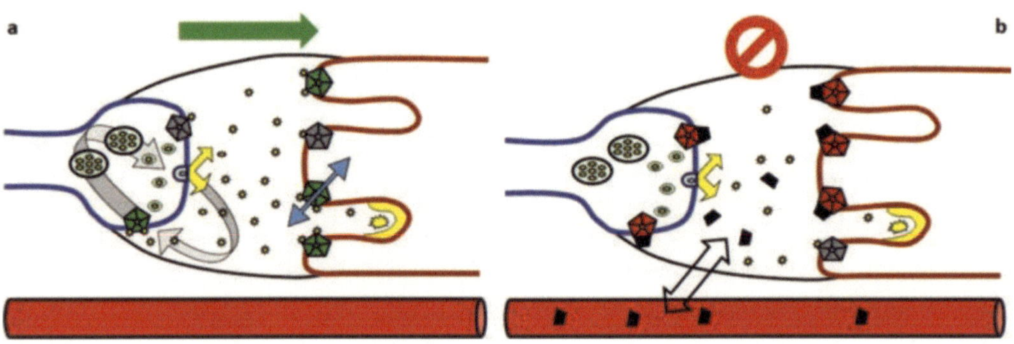


**Figure 2.** Neuromuscular transmission (a) and blockade (b). (a) The motor nerve (on the left) synthetizes, stores, and liberates vesicles of acetylcholine in the synaptic cleft when it depolarizes. Acetylcholines (*yellow stars*) bind to postsynaptic nicotinic receptors to open the ionic channel and depolarize the muscle membrane (on the right), inducing the muscle contraction. Cholinesterases inactivate rapidly acetylcholine in the folds of the motor end plate. Presynaptic nicotinic receptors allow for a positive feedback on the nerve in order to liberate more acetylcholine to induce intense contraction. (b) Neuromuscular blocking agents (*black trapezes*) distribute from the plasma into the synaptic cleft to bind and inactivate the nicotinic receptors on pre- and postsynaptic membranes, competitively with acetylcholine.

Non-depolarizing neuromuscular blocking agents (NMBA) fix competitively with ACh on nicotinic receptors. On presynaptic receptors, for which they have the highest affinity, they prevent the mobilization and release of storages of ACh, inducing fade to repetitive nerve stimulation because of a lack of available ACh. On the postsynaptic receptors, they prevent the membrane from depolarizing and, therefore, initiating the muscle contraction. The NMB is a combination of these two actions (**Figure 2b**).

http://dx.doi.org/10.5772/64934

According to the pharmacokinetics of each drug, NMBA is metabolized and/or progressively eliminated from the plasma. The concentration decreases in the synaptic cleft and, as ACh can reach more and more receptors, the neuromuscular transmission (NMT) recovers gradually.

During anesthesia, the level of NMB can be monitored with the use of a nerve stimulator (**Figure 3**). As the standard, the ulnar nerve is stimulated at the wrist and the degree of relaxation is measured at the adductor pollicis muscle [48]. The motor nerve is stimulated by standardized electric patterns:

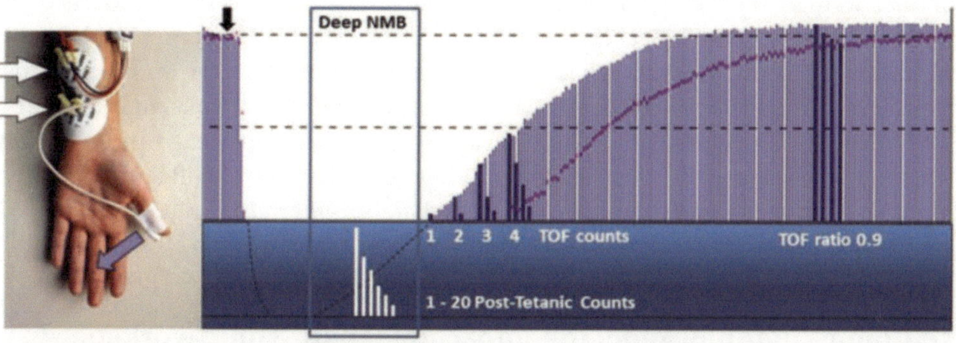


**Figure 3.** Neuromuscular transmission monitoring. The ulnar nerve is electrically stimulated at the wrist by train of four (TOF) or post-tetanic count (PTC) sequences. The thumb movements are recorded and displayed during the onset (after neuromuscular blocking agent administration: black arrow) and spontaneous recovery of a neuromuscular blockade: vertical lines represent the first twitch height (T1), purple dots are the TOF ratio (T4/T1), PTC and TOF count are additionally represented. Deep neuromuscular blockade is defined as TOF count 0 and PTC ≥ 1.

- The train-of-four (TOF) [49] is an automatic repetition of four square electric twitches (200 μs) at 2 Hz for every 15 s. The current intensity can be set according to every patient characteristic (50–60 mA as the default level). During NMB recovery and related to presynaptic fade, TOF recovers progressively 1, 2, 3, and then 4 counts before a TOF ratio (relative height of T4/T1) can quantify the residual fade until reaching 1.
- When there is no response to TOF, the post-tetanic count (PTC) [50] is another automatic sequence dedicated to monitoring deeper levels of blockade, including a tetanic stimulation (twitches at 50–100 Hz during 5 s) to mobilize presynaptic storages of ACh before 20 single twitches (1 Hz) are delivered.

The corresponding muscle responses are evaluated by the operator (visual or tactile subjective evaluation) or, much better, are objectively quantified by a dedicated monitor. Then, the complete course of any NMB can be accurately described by PTC, TOF count, and TOF ratio. Unfortunately, many clinicians still do not use objective monitors in their clinical practice [51]. This is undoubtedly a prerequisite to proper intraoperative management of NMB.

According to PTC, TOF count, and TOF ratio, different levels of NMB are determined as follows: [31, 48]

- Intense block: no response to PTC.
- Deep NMB: a PTC one or more but no response to TOF.
- Moderate block: TOF count 1–3.
- Shallow block: a TOF count of 4 with fade, quantified as TOF ratio.
- Threshold for safe tracheal extubation: TOF ratio >0.9.

It is important to know that different muscle groups have different sensitivities to NMBAs [52, 53]. Particularly, the adductor pollicis muscle is more sensitive to NMBAs compared with the abdominal wall muscles and the diaphragm, which have a more rapid recovery [54–56]. Consequently, the depth of blockade at the thumb does not reflect the exact level of blockade at the other muscle groups. Even when no TOF count is recorded at the thumb, laparoscopic surgeons may experience insufficient relaxation of the abdominal wall muscles that could induce unexpected movements of the IA instruments and could impair the surgical conditions. On the other hand, using PTC allows for properly monitoring deep NMB at the thumb and is sufficiently sensitive to ensure enough diaphragm paralysis for most clinical purposes [57, 58].

## 4. Neuromuscular blockade: the impact on laparoscopic workspace

Modern anesthesia provides every patient undergoing laparoscopic surgery with a combination of drugs and techniques as closely adapted to his physical status as possible, including hypnotic agents, multimodal analgesia, lung ventilation in head-down position, hemodynamic and fluid management, and postoperative nausea prevention. Among them, NMB is indicated for intubation and during the surgical procedure. But, as do most drugs, NMBAs have some risks related to their administration, including:

- Anaphylaxis (1/13,000, depending on the drug). Anesthesiologists are trained to manage this acute complication (protocol, algorithm, and simulation).
- Awareness during the procedure. Monitoring of the depth of anesthesia continues to improve, including using the bispectral index, which helps to prevent awareness during anesthesia [59].
- Residual paralysis at the time of tracheal extubation (see Section 5).

As a consequence, some anesthesiologists might be reluctant to induce deep NMB, especially during the entire procedure. Satisfactory surgical conditions are the end product of multiple factors that may range from the level of general anesthesia administered to the skill of the surgeon and the collaboration between the surgeon and the anesthesiologist [60]. In clinical practice, when a surgeon experiences surgical conditions that are less than satisfactory, the anesthesiologist can take some of the following actions [61]:

- Changing the body position.

- Increasing the depth of anesthesia (high dose of hypnotics, vapors, and/or opioids).
- Changing the ventilator patterns.
- Increasing the insufflation pressure.

These alternatives often cause cardiovascular depression and increased peak airway pressure and cannot reliably abolish all movements [62, 63]. Without appropriate NMB, sudden muscle contractions are experienced in ±30% of laparoscopic procedures [64, 65]. The initial (blind) insertion of the trocars is a high-risk part of the laparoscopic procedure that could cause the most serious complications related to laparoscopy, such as perforations of a bowel or a large vessel [66]. The establishment of a deep NMB in this initial part of the procedure seems to be essential to reduce the possible occurrence of these complications. However, no study actually demonstrates that maintaining a deep NMB reduces the surgical complication rate [60], and NMB should not be used as a substitute for adequate depth of anesthesia [31].

Ultimately, what level of NMB is associated with optimal conditions for laparoscopic surgery, and does a deep NMB provide superior operating conditions for laparoscopy than does a moderate block?

### 4.1. Studies to determine the interest of deep NMB during pelvic laparoscopy

The requirement for muscle relaxation has evolved with the development of surgery. Few studies addressed this question in the specific field of gynecologic laparoscopy. Different methods were used, making comparison difficult and inducing a risk of bias in the interpretation of the results. The most frequent outcome was the subjective surgeon's assessment of the surgical conditions during the procedure [61]. Different surgical rating scales (SRSs) (three to five points) were used to quantify the quality of the surgical field and the operating conditions, ranging from excellent to poor or unacceptable. However, these scales have not yet been validated for assessment of surgical conditions.

To enable the reader to come to his own conclusion, the different studies available in pelvic/gynecological laparoscopic surgery are summarized in **Table 1** given below [65, 67–73].

| **Authors, year, reference**<br>**Type of surgery, n** | **NMB design**<br>**Method of evaluation** | **Relevant results concerning surgical conditions** |
|---|---|---|
| Bertrand et al. (1983) [67]<br>Various gynecological lap, $n = 40$ | Succinylcholine 1 mg $kg^{-1}$ + infusion or vecuronium 0.05–0.06–0.07 mg $kg^{-1}$<br>SRS 4 grades | Better muscle relaxation, less supplemental vecuronium and less IAP with succinylcholine or 0.07 mg $kg^{-1}$ vecuronium. |
| Swann et al. (1993) [68]<br>Various gynecological lap, $n = 60$ | Atracurium 0.3 mg $kg^{-1}$ (TT) versus no NMB (LMA).<br>SRS 3 grades | Two poor conditions in the no NMB group (vs 0 in Atracurium group), but concluded as not clinically different. |

| Authors, year, reference<br>Type of surgery, n | NMB design<br>Method of evaluation | Relevant results concerning surgical conditions |
|---|---|---|
| Chassard et al. (1996) [69]<br>Various gynecological lap,<br>$n = 50$ | Atracurium 0.25 mg $kg^{-1}$ + boluses to maintain T1 < 10% versus no NMB.<br>SRS 4 grades | The operating conditions were not influenced by NMB. |
| Williams et al. (2003) [70]<br>Day case gynecological lap,<br>$n = 40$ | Atracurium 0.5 mg/kg (TT) supple mented as required, versus no NMB (LMA).<br>SRS 4 grades | Better adequacy of pneumoperitoneum with NMB; 28% inadequate trocar insertion in the no NMB group |
| Paek et al. (2009) [71]<br>Pelvic laparoscopy,<br>$n = 56$ | Rocuronium 0.6 mg $kg^{-1}$ + 0.15 mg $kg^{-1}$ boluses to maintain TOF count ≤ 2 versus no additional bolus.<br>Events, IAP | No coughing, bucking or movement during procedures.<br>No supplemental NMBA required during propofol remifentanil anesthesia. |
| Chen et al. (2013) [72]<br>Gynecological lap,<br>$n = 120$ | Rocuronium 0.6 mg $kg^{-1}$ versus no NMB. LMA in all cases.<br>Surgeon's questionnaire | Comparable surgical conditions. No benefit of NMB during anesthesia with LMA. |
| Dubois et al. (2014) [65]<br>Lap hysterectomy,<br>$n = 100$ | Rocuronium 0.6 mg $kg^{-1}$ + 5 mg boluses to maintain TOF count ≤ 2 versus shallower NMB.<br>SRS 4 grades | Deep NMB provided better (excellent) surgical conditions when TOF count = 0 and prevented unacceptable conditions (28% in shallow NMB). |
| Madsen et al. (2015) [73]<br>Gynecologic lap,<br>$n = 14$ | Rocuronium 1 mg $kg^{-1}$ deep NMB versus no NMB.<br>SRS 4 grades<br>Distance from sacral promontory to the trocar | Slightly improved workspace and better conditions during suturing of the fascia with deep NMB. |

**Table 1.** Studies investigating the interest of neuromuscular blockade during gynecological laparoscopic surgery.

Overall, there is good evidence that NMB optimizes surgical conditions in gynecological laparoscopy. This was also true during laparoscopic prostatectomy and nephrectomy. Deep NMB seems superior to moderate NMB [61, 74, 75].

In addition, when compared to moderate NMB (or no NMB) during upper abdominal laparoscopy, deep NMB marginally optimizes surgical conditions and allows the IAB pressure to be reduced by 3–5 mmHg without compromising surgical conditions [61, 76].

It seems useful to establish a deep NMB from the beginning of the procedure instead of waiting for the surgeon to request it [46]. The main problem is the residual block at the end of surgery and the time needed to recover before being able to extubate the patient. This issue is addressed in the following section.

## 5. The residual neuromuscular blockade after surgery

Any administration of a NMBA during general anesthesia carries the risk of residual effects after surgery. This becomes inevitable when maintaining the NMB deep until the end of the surgical procedure. Based on numerous studies, postoperative residual NMB is defined as a TOF ratio <0.9 [77, 78]. Its incidence when arriving in the post-anesthesia care unit (PACU) is estimated to be approximately 40% of the patients who received NMBA in clinical practice. Residual NMB has clinical consequences and complications that can prolong hospitalization. Before reaching the safety threshold of TOF ratio >0.9, the most frequent adverse events include patient anxiety, upper airway collapse because of the high sensitivity of pharyngeal muscles to NMBA [79], hypoxia because of the decreased sensitivity of chemoreceptors [80], and dysphagia and reduced protection against aspiration increasing the risk of postoperative pneumonia [81]. For these reasons, guidelines should be observed to rule out any level of residual NMB before awakening and extubating the patient. Current recommendations are to use short- or intermediate-acting NMBAs, to routinely reverse all NMB, and to monitor neuromuscular transmission whenever relaxants are used, especially before and after NMB reversal [82–84]. By decreasing the incidence of the residual NMB in the PACU, patient safety is improved, as is demonstrated by the reduction in postoperative respiratory complications [85].

### 5.1. Quantitative neuromuscular transmission monitoring in daily practice

The use of neuromuscular transmission (NMT) monitoring is mandatory to manage deep NMB and to determine the threshold for the administration of the appropriate doses of reversal agents and, finally, to confirm their effect until attaining a TOF ratio >0.9. Unfortunately, visual or manual evaluation of the contraction intensity induced by the nerve stimulation does not allow for the effective quantification of the relative force of the successive muscular responses and, consequently, lacks accuracy and cannot exclude significant levels of residual NMB [86]. The recommendation is to use objective measures to confirm NMB recovery at a minimum of a TOF ratio of 0.9 before extubating the patient [83]. Measurements obtained by recording techniques (i.e., the application of custom sensors) using the principles of acceleromyography, kinemyography, or electromyography have proved their effectiveness, with some specific precautions [82, 87–89]. Implementing these quantitative monitors to manage every NMBA administration in daily practice demonstrated a reduction in the residual NMB incidence to a very low level [90].

### 5.2. Pharmacological reversal of the residual NMB

- Neostigmine antagonizes a non-depolarizing NMB by increasing the availability of acetylcholine (ACh) in the synaptic cleft, tipping the competitive balance in favor of the neurotransmitter primarily by inactivating the acetylcholinesterases at the muscle endplate (**Figure 4a**).

Administered routinely at the end of anesthesia, neostigmine has demonstrated a positive effect on postoperative mortality [91]. Beyond this favorable overall trend, the effectiveness of NMB reversal with neostigmine is limited by several specific problems.

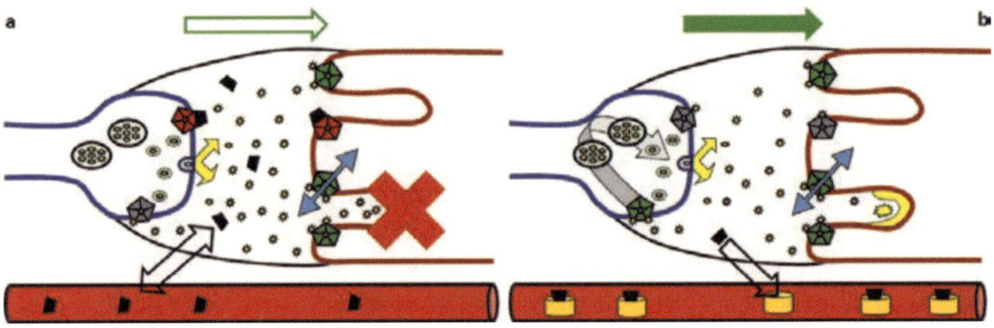


**Figure 4.** Reversal agents. (a) Neostigmine inhibits cholinesterase making more acetylcholine available in the synaptic cleft. The competitive block evolves in favor of the acetylcholine and neuromuscular transmission increases gradually. Neuromuscular blocking agents still present are progressively eliminated according to their pharmacokinetic properties. (b) Sugammadex encapsulates rocuronium in the plasma, washing the synaptic cleft of all neuromuscular blocking agents for good. Normal neuromuscular transmission recovers rapidly.

Even the maximal recommended dose of 70 μg/kg (or 5 mg) has limited effects and cannot effectively reverse deep levels of NMB [92]. Neostigmine can only be administered from a moderate block with a minimum TOF of 3 to increase efficacy and safety [93, 94]. Moreover, the delay needed for reversal with neostigmine (10–15 min on average) has a large interindividual variability. Patients might need more than 60 min to reach a TOF ratio of 0.9 [95]. The problem is that most anesthesiologists will not wait long enough before extubating their patients. Consequently, even when routinely administered, neostigmine is frequently insufficient to completely reverse the residual NMB at the time of tracheal extubation [96]. The risk of residual blockade without quantitative NMT monitors is significant. Even when using a peripheral nerve stimulator with subjective (visual or tactile) evaluation, more than 50% of the patients could experience residual NMB after the administration of neostigmine [97]. Then, only the proper use of neostigmine guided by NMT monitors can help eliminate postoperative respiratory complications associated with the use of NMBA [82, 83, 98].

Because neostigmine is an acetylcholinesterase inhibitor, it induces ACh stimulation on muscarinic receptors in smooth muscles, the heart and various glands and nicotinic receptors in the autonomic ganglia, which induce adverse side effects including postoperative nausea and/or vomiting, bradycardia, prolonged QT interval, unpredictable bronchoconstriction, ptyalism, and increased intraluminal pressure and propulsive activity in the bowels [99]. To

http://dx.doi.org/10.5772/64934

prevent some of these side effects, parasympathicolytic drugs (atropine or glycopyrrolate) are administered simultaneously. These compounds are also accompanied by potential secondary effects (i.e., tachycardia, urinary retention, accommodation disorders, and dry mouth).

Because of the limited ability of anticholinesterases to antagonize deep NMB, most clinicians wisely attempt to avoid deep block as the end of surgery approaches, exposing the surgeon and the patient to impaired surgical conditions. But recently with the availability of sugammadex as an alternative to neostigmine, there has been renewed interest in other potential indications for the intraoperative maintenance of deep NMB, especially for laparoscopic surgery [31].

- Sugammadex is a selective relaxant-binding agent [100]. The modified gamma-cyclodextrin encapsulates the steroidal NMBAs rocuronium or vecuronium present in the plasma and the neuromuscular synaptic cleft. The concentration of the free steroidal NMBA is rapidly reduced. The nicotinergic receptors again become available to ACh, and the NMB fades rapidly (**Figure 4b**). The steroidal NMBA-sugammadex complexes remain bound until they are excreted by the kidneys. Because of the molecular selectivity for steroidal NMBAs, sugammadex has no effect on the benzylisoquinolines (atracurium, cisatracurium, and mivacurium).

Different doses of sugammadex have been determined to guarantee effective reversal according to the depth of the NMB (according to the plasma concentration of the steroidal NMBA) [101]. A dose of 4 mg/kg is indicated to reverse deep NMB within a few minutes (**Figure 5**). It is not only much faster and more predictable than neostigmine, but it is also able to reverse all depths of blockades [95, 101]. In addition, sugammadex has an excellent clinical tolerance, few side effects, and it is beneficial for numerous categories of patients who are at a particular risk for developing complications from residual NMB or for undesirable effects from neostigmine [45, 101].

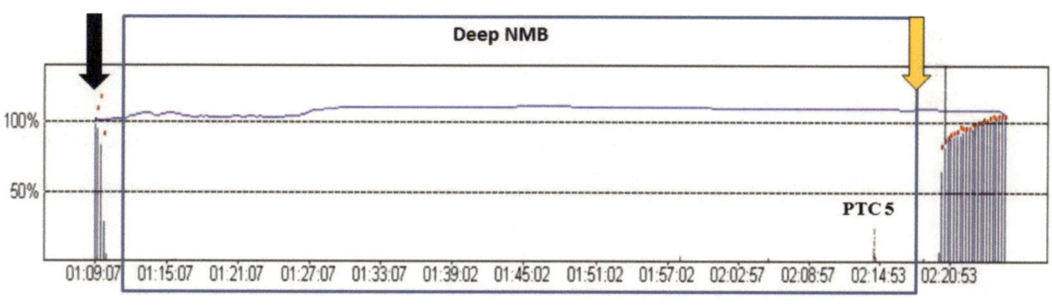


**Figure 5.** Deep NMB during the entire laparoscopic procedure. Following rocuronium administration (*black arrow*), a deep neuromuscular blockade is maintained until the end of surgery. Then, sugammadex (*orange arrow*) allowed for a fast and complete reversal.

As an innovative drug, sugammadex is expensive when compared with most drugs used in anesthesia. Intraoperative maintenance of deep NMB and sugammadex reversal have important economic repercussions that could call into question the routine use of deep NMB for laparoscopic surgery [60]. On the other hand, every minute of open operating theater time has a high financial value [102]. A few minutes spared with a faster and more predictable reversal strategy allowing for a shorter operating room discharge can balance the cost of the new drug and contribute to optimization of operating theater turnover and overall financial return [103].

## 6. Conclusion

The introduction of sugammadex into clinical practice provides the opportunity to modify the management of NMB to improve the surgical conditions during laparoscopy as well as the safety of the patients. The maintenance of a deep rocuronium induced NMB from the trocar insertion until the end of laparoscopy is no longer incompatible with rapid recovery and awakening in optimal conditions. In all cases, NMT monitoring is the key to adequate NMB management. Objective measurements allow for excellent intubation and surgical conditions, the definition of thresholds and doses for the administration of reversal agents, and the exclusion of residual NMB prior to the patient extubation.

## Author details

Christophe Dransart, Laurie Putz, Maria-Laura Marotta and Philippe E. Dubois*

*Address all correspondence to: phil.dubois@uclouvain.be

CHU UCL Namur, Yvoir, Belgium

## References

[1] Hatzinger M et al. Hans Christian Jacobaeus: inventor of human laparoscopy and thoracoscopy. J Endourol 2006; 20: 848–850.

[2] Litynski GS. Raoul Palmer, World War II, and transabdominal coelioscopy. Laparoscopy extends into gynecology. JSLS 1997; 1: 289–92.

[3] Hurd W et al. "Gynecologic Laparoscopy"; Medscape: http://emedicine.medscape.com/article/265201; updated in 28 December 2015.

[4] Bosteels J et al. The effectiveness of reproductive surgery in the treatment of female infertility: facts, views and vision. Facts Views Vis Obgyn 2010; 2: 232–52.

[5] Bosteels J et al. The position of diagnostic laparoscopy in current fertility practice. Hum Reprod Update 2007; 13: 477–85.

[6] Practice Committee of the American Society for Reproductive Medicine. Diagnostic evaluation of the infertile female: a committee opinion. Fertil Steril 2015; 103: 44–50.

[7] Practice Committee of the American Society for Reproductive Medicine. Role of tubal surgery in the era of assisted reproductive technology: a committee opinion. Fertil Steril 2015; 103: 37–43.

[8] Gala RB, Society of Gynecologic Surgeons Systematic Review Group. Systematic review of robotic surgery in gynecology: robotic techniques compared with laparoscopy and laparotomy. J Minim Invasive Gynecol 2014; 21: 353–61.

[9] Kim SM et al. Abdominal, multi-port and single-port total laparoscopic hysterectomy: eleven-year trends comparison of surgical outcomes complications of 936 cases. Arch Gynecol Obstet 2015; 291: 1313–9.

[10] Zhao M et al. Single-incision multiport laparoscopy versus multichannel-tipped single port laparoscopy in gynecologic surgery: outcomes and benefits. Int J Clin Exp Med 2015; 8: 14992–8.

[11] Park JY et al. Laparoendoscopic single-site compared with conventional laparoscopic ovarian cystectomy for ovarian endometrioma. J Minim Invasive Gynecol 2015; 22: 813–9.

[12] Donnez J, Dolmans MM. Uterine fibroid management: from the present to the future. Hum Reprod Update. 2016 Jul 27. [Epub ahead of print]

[13] Malbrain M, De Laet I, De Waele J et al. The role of abdominal compliance, the neglected parameter in critically ill patients—a consensus review of 16. Part 2: measurement techniques and management recommandations. Anaesthesiol Intensive Ther 2014; 46: 406–32.

[14] Mulier J, Dillemans B, Van Cauwenberge S. Impact of the patient's body position on the intraabdominal workspace during laparoscopic surgery. Surg Endosc. 2010; 24: 1398–1402.

[15] Mulier J, Dillemans B, Crombach M et al. On the abdominal pressure volume relationship. Internet J Anesthesiol 2008; 21 :1–7.

[16] Hypolito OH et al. Creation of pneumoperitoneum: noninvasive monitoring of clinical effects of elevated intraperitoneal pressure for the insertion of the first trocar. Surg Endosc 2010; 24: 1663–1669.

[17] Özdemir-van Brunschot D et al. What is the evidence for the use of low-pressure pneumoperitoneum? A systematic review. Surg Endosc 2016; 30: 2049–2065.

[18] Strang CM, Freden F, Maripuu E et al. Improved ventilation-perfusion matching with increasing abdominal pressure during $CO_2$-pneumoperitoneum in pigs. Acta Anaesthesiol Scand 2011; 55: 887–96.

[19] Dexter SP, Vucevic M, Gibson J, McMahon MJ. Hemodynamic consequences of high- and low-pressure capnoperitoneum during laparoscopic cholecystectomy. Surg Endosc 1999; 13: 376–81.

[20] Matsuzaki S et al. Impact of intraperitoneal pressure of a $CO_2$ pneumoperitoneum on the surgical peritoneal environment. Hum Reprod 2012; 27: 1613–1623.

[21] Schietroma M et al. Changes in the blood coagulation, fibrinolysis, and cytokine profile during laparoscopic and open cholecystectomy. Surg Endosc 2004; 18: 1090–1096.

[22] Gurusamy KS, Samraj K, Davidson BR. Low pressure versus standard pressure pneumoperitoneum in laparoscopic cholecystectomy. Cochrane Database Syst Rev 2009; 2: CD006930.

[23] Barczyński M, Herman RM. A prospective randomized trial on comparison of low-pressure (LP) and standard-pressure (SP) pneumoperitoneum for laparoscopic cholecystectomy. Surg Endosc 2003; 17: 533–8.

[24] Joshipura VP, Haribhakti SP, Patel N et al. A prospective randomized, controlled study comparing low pressure versus high pressure pneumoperitoneum during laparoscopic cholecystectomy. Surg Laparosc Endosc Percutan Tech 2009; 19: 234–40.

[25] Sarli L, Costi R, Sansebastiano G, Trivelli M, Roncoroni L. Prospective randomized trial of low-pressure pneumoperitoneum for reduction of shoulder-tip pain following laparoscopy. Br J Surg 2000; 87: 1161–5.

[26] Kandil TS, El Hefnawy E. Shoulder pain following laparoscopic cholecystectomy: factors affecting the incidence and severity. J Laparoendosc Adv Surg Tech 2010; 20: 677–82.

[27] Yasir M, Mehta KS, Banday VH et al. Evaluation of postoperative shoulder tip pain in low pressure versus standard pressure pneumoperitoneum during laparoscopic .cholecystectomy. Surgeon 2012; 10: 71–4.

[28] Bogani G et al. Low vs standard pneumoperitoneum pressure during laparoscopic hysterectomy: prospective randomized trial. J Minim Invasive Gynecol 2014; 21: 466–471.

[29] Topcu HO et al. A prospective randomized trial of postoperative pain following different insufflation pressures during gynecologic laparoscopy. Eur J Obstet Gynecol Reprod Biol 2014; 182: 81–85.

[30] Radosa JC, Radosa MP, Mavrova R et al. Five minutes of extended assisted ventilation with an open umbilical trocar valve significantly reduces postoperative abdominal and shoulder pain in patients undergoing laparoscopic hysterectomy. Eur J Obstet Gynecol Reprod Biol 2013; 171: 122–7.

[31] Kopman A, Naguib M. Laparoscopic surgery and muscle relaxants: is deep block helpful? Anesth Analg. 2015; 120: 51–58.

[32] Hua J, Gong J, Yao L, Zhou B, Song Z. Low-pressure versus standard-pressure pneumoperitoneum for laparoscopic cholecystectomy: a systematic review and meta-analysis. Am J Surg 2014; 208: 143–50.

[33] Mouton WG, Bessell JR, Otten KT, Maddern GJ. Pain after laparoscopy. Surg Endosc 1999; 13: 445–8.

[34] Donatsky AM, Bjerrum F, Gogenur I. Surgical techniques to minimize shoulder pain after laparoscopic cholecystectomy. A systematic review. Surg Endosc 2013; 27: 2275–2282.

[35] Vijayaraghavan N, Sistla SC, Kundra P et al. Comparison of standard-pressure and low-pressure pneumoperitoneum in laparoscopic cholecystectomy: a double blinded randomized controlled study. Surg Laparosc Endosc Percutan Tech 2014; 24: 127–33.

[36] Gurusamy KS, Vaughan J, Davidson BR. Low pressure versus standard pressure pneumoperitoneum in laparoscopic cholecystectomy. Cochrane Database Syst Rev 2014; (3): CD006930.

[37] Warlé MC, Berkers AW, Langenhuijsen JF et al. Low-pressure pneumoperitoneum during laparoscopic donor nephrectomy to optimize live donors' comfort. Clin Transplant 2013; 27: E478–83.

[38] Cravello L et al. Laparoscopic surgery in gynecology: randomized prospective study comparing pneumoperitoneum and abdominal wall suspension. Eur J Obstet Gynecol Reprod Biol 1999; 83: 9–14.

[39] Neudecker J et al. The European Association for Endoscopic Surgery clinical practice guideline on the pneumoperitoneum for laparoscopic surgery. Surg Endosc 2002; 16: 1121–1143.

[40] Staehr-Rye A, Rasmussen L, Rosenberg J et al. Surgical space conditions during low-pressure laparoscopic cholecystectomy with deep versus moderate neuromuscular blockade: a randomized clinical study. Anesthesia Analgesia 2014; 119: 1084–92.

[41] Griffith HR, Johnson GE. The use of curare in general anesthesia. Anesthesiology 1942; 3: 418–420.

[42] Gray TC, Halton J. Technique for the use of d-tubocurarine chloride with balanced anaesthesia. BMJ 1946; 2: 293–295.

[43] Beecher HK, Todd DP. A study of the deaths associated with anesthesia and surgery. Ann Surg 1954; 140: 2–34.

[44] Mencke T, Echternach M, Kleinschmidt S et al. Laryngeal morbidity and quality of tracheal intubation: a randomized controlled trial. Anesthesiology 2003; 98: 1049–56.

[45] Dubois PE, Mulier JP. A review of the interest of sugammadex for deep neuromuscular blockade management in Belgium. Acta Anaesthesiol Belg 2013; 64: 49–60.

[46] Madsen M, Staehr-Rye A, Claudius C, Gatke M. Is deep neuromuscular blockade beneficial in laparoscopic surgery? Yes, probably. Acta Anaesthesiol Scand 2016; 60: 710–6.

[47] Fagerlund MJ, Eriksson LI. Current concept in neuromuscular transmission. Br J Anaesth 2009; 103: 108–14.

[48] Fuchs-Buder T, Claudius C, Skovgaard LT et al. Good clinical research practice in pharmacodynamic studies of neuromuscular blocking agents II: the Stockholm revision. Acta Anaesthesiol Scand 2007; 51:789–808.

[49] Ali HH, Utting JE, Gray C. Stimulus frequency in the detection of neuromuscular block in humans. Br J Anaesth 1970; 42: 967–78.

[50] Viby-Mogensen J et al. Posttetanic count (PTC): a new method of evaluating an intense nondepolarizing neuromuscular blockade. Anesthesiology 1981; 55: 458–61.

[51] Naguib M, Kopman AF, Lien CA et al. A survey of current management of neuromuscular block in the United States and Europe. Anesth Analg 2010; 111: 11–9.

[52] Meistelman C, Plaud B, Donati F. Rocuronium neuromuscular blockade at the adductor muscles of the larynx and adductor pollicis in humans. Can J Anaesth 1992; 39: 665–9.

[53] Hemmerling TM, Donati F. Neuromuscular blockade at the larynx, the diaphragm and the corrugator supercilii muscle: a review. Can J Anaesth 2003; 50: 779–94.

[54] Cantineau JP, Porte F, d'Honneur G, Duvaldestin P. Neuromuscular effects of rocuronium on the diaphragm and adductor pollicis muscles in anesthetized patients. Anesthesiology 1994; 81: 585–90.

[55] Kirov K, Motamed C, Dhonneur G. Differential sensitivity of abdominal muscles and the diaphragm to mivacurium: an electromyographic study. Anesthesiology 2001; 95: 1323–8.

[56] Moerer O, Baller C, Hinz J et al. Neuromuscular effects of rapacuronium on the diaphragm and skeletal muscles in anaesthetized patients using cervical magnetic stimulation for stimulating the phrenic nerves. Eur J Anaesthesiol 2002; 19: 883–7.

[57] Fernando PU, Viby-Mogensen J, Bonsu AK et al. Relationship between posttetanic count and response to carinal stimulation during vecuronium-induced neuromuscular blockade. Acta Anaesthesiol Scand 1987; 31: 593–6.

[58] Dhonneur G, Kirov K, Motamed C et al. Post-tetanic count at adductor pollicis is a better indicator of early diaphragmatic recovery than train-of-four count at corrugator supercilii. Br J Anaesth 2007; 99: 376–379.

[59] Myles PS, Leslie K, McNeil J et al. Bispectral index monitoring to prevent awareness during anaesthesia: the B-Aware randomised controlled trial. Lancet 2004; 363: 1757–63.

[60] Kopman AF, Naguib M. Is deep neuromuscular block beneficial in laparoscopic surgery? No, probably not. Acta Anaesthesiol Scand 2016; 60: 717–22.

[61] Madsen M, Staehr-Rye AK, Gätke MR, Claudius C. Neuromuscular blockade for optimising surgical conditions during abdominal and gynaecological surgery: a systematic review. Acta Anaesthesiol Scand 2015; 59: 1–16.

[62] Maurtua MA, Deogaonkar A, Bakri MH et al. Dosing of remifentanil to prevent movement during craniotomy in the absence of neuromuscular blockade. J Neurosurg Anesthesiol 2008; 20: 221–5.

[63] Green RS, Edwards J, Sabri E, Fergusson D. Evaluation of the incidence, risk factors, and impact on patient outcomes of postintubation hemodynamic instability. CJEM 2012; 14: 74–82.

[64] Blobner M, Frick CG, Stäuble RB et al. Neuromuscular blockade improves surgical conditions. Surg Endosc 2015; 29: 627–36.

[65] Dubois PE, Putz L, Jamart J et al. Deep neuromuscular block improves surgical conditions during laparoscopic hysterectomy: a randomised controlled trial. Eur J Anaesthesiol 2014; 31: 1–7.

[66] Ahmad G, O'Flynn H, Duffy JM, Phillips K, Watson A. Laparoscopic entry techniques. Cochrane Database Syst Rev 2012; 2: CD006583.

[67] Bertrand M, Lienhart A, Daloz M et al. Clinical use of vecuronium during celioscopy. Ann Fr Anesth Reanim 1983; 2: 27–31.

[68] Swann DG, Spens H, Edwards SA, Chestnut RJ. Anaesthesia for gynaecological laparoscopy -a comparison between the laryngeal mask airway and tracheal intubation. Anaesthesia 1993; 48: 431–434.

[69] Chassard D, Bryssine B, Golfier F et al. Gynecologic laparoscopy with or without curare. Ann Fr Anesth Reanim 1996; 15: 1013–1017.

[70] Williams MT, Rice I, Ewen SP, Elliott SM. A comparison of the effect of two anaesthetic techniques on surgical conditions during gynaecological laparoscopy. Anaesthesia 2003; 58: 574–578.

[71] Paek CM, Yi JW, Lee BJ, Kang JM. No supplemental muscle relaxants are required during propofol and remifentanil total intravenous anesthesia for laparoscopic pelvic surgery. J Laparoendosc Adv Surg Tech A 2009; 19: 33–7.

[72] Chen BZ, Tan L, Zhang L, Shang YC. Is muscle relaxant necessary in patients undergoing laparoscopic gynecological surgery with a ProSeal LMA? J Clin Anesth 2013; 25: 32–35.

[73] Madsen MV, Gätke MR, Springborg HH et al. Optimising abdominal space with deep neuromuscular blockade in gynaecologic laparoscopy– a randomised blinded cross-over study. Acta Anaesthesiol Scand 2015; 59: 441–7.

[74] Martini CH, Boon M, Bevers RF et al. Evaluation of surgical conditions during laparoscopic surgery in patients with moderate vs deep neuromuscular block. Br J Anaesth 2014; 112: 498–505.

[75] Dubois PE. TOF count 0 ensured optimal surgical conditions during laparoscopic hysterectomy. Eur J Anaesthesiol. 2015; 32: 65–6.

[76] Van Wijk RM, Watts RW, Ledowski T, Trochsler M, Moran JL, Arenas GWN. Deep neuromuscular block reduces intra-abdominal pressure requirements during laparoscopic cholecystectomy: a prospective observational study. Acta Anaesthesiol Scand 2015; 59: 434–40.

[77] Plaud B et al. Residual paralysis after emergence from anaesthesia. Anesthesiology 2010; 112: 1013–2.

[78] Murphy GS, Brull SJ. Residual neuromuscular block: lessons unlearned. Part I: definitions, incidence, and adverse physiologic effects of residual neuromuscular block. Anesth Analg 2010; 111: 120–8.

[79] Eriksson LI et al. Functionnal assessment of the pharynx at rest and during swallowing in partially paralysed humans. Anesthesiology 1997; 87: 1035–43.

[80] Eriksson LI et al. Attenuated ventilatory response to hypoxemia at vecuronium-induced partial neuromuscular block. Acta Anesthesiol Scand 1992; 36: 710–5.

[81] Berg H. Viby-Mogensen J et al. Residual neuromuscular block is a risk factor for postoperative pulmonary complications. Acta Anesthesiol Scand 1997; 41: 1095–1103.

[82] Murphy GS, Brull SJ. Residual neuromuscular block: lessons unlearned. Part II: methods to reduce the risk of residual weakness. Anesth Analg 2010; 111: 129–40.

[83] Viby-Mogensen J, Claudius C. Evidence-based management of neuromuscular Block. Anesth Analg 2010; 111: 1–2.

[84] Miller RD, Ward TA. Monitoring and pharmacologic reversal of a nondepolarizing neuromuscular blockade should be routine. Anesth Analg 2010; 111: 3–5.

[85] Murphy GS, Szokol JW, Avram MJ et al. Intraoperative acceleromyography monitoring reduces symptoms of muscle weakness and improves quality of recovery in the early postoperative period. Anesthesiology 2011; 115: 946–54.

[86] Cammu G, De Witte J, De Veylder J et al. Postoperative residual paralysis in outpatients versus inpatients. Anesth Analg 2006; 102: 426–9.

[87] Claudius C, Viby-Mogensen J. Acceleromyography for use in scientific and clinical practice. A systematic review of the evidence. Anesthesiology 2008; 108: 1117–40.

[88] Murphy GS, Szokol JW, Marymont JH et al. Intraoperative acceleromyographic monitoring reduces the risk of residual neuromuscular blockade and adverse respiratory events in the postanesthesia care unit. Anesthesiology 2008; 109: 389–99.

[89] Dubois PE, De Bel M, Jamart J et al. Performance of acceleromyography with a short and light TOF-tube compared with mechanomyography. A clinical comparison. Eur J Anaesthesiol. 2014; 31: 404–10.

[90] Baillard et al. Postoperative residual neuromuscular block: a survey of management. Br J Anaesth 2005; 95: 622–6.

[91] Arbous MS, Meursing AE, van Kleef JW et al. Impact of anesthesia management characteristics on severe morbidity and mortality. Anesthesiology 2005; 102: 257–68.

[92] Bartkowsky RR. Incomplete reversal of pancuronium neuromuscular blockade by neostigmine, pyridostigmine and edrophonium. Anesth Analg 1987; 66: 594–598.

[93] Kirkegaard H, Heier T, Caldwell JE. Efficacy of tactile-guided reversal from cisatracurium-induced neuromuscular block. Anesthesiology 2002; 96: 45–50.

[94] Srivastava A, Hunter JM. Reversal of neuromuscular block. Br J Anaesth 2009; 103: 115–29.

[95] Blobner M, Eriksson LI, Scholz J et al. Reversal of rocuronium-induced neuromuscular blockade with sugammadex compared with neostigmine during sevoflurane anaesthesia: results of a randomised, controlled trial. Eur J Anaesthesiol 2010; 27: 874–881.

[96] Murphy GS, Szokol JW, Marymont JH et al. Residual paralysis at the time of tracheal extubation. Anesth Analg 2005; 100: 1840–5.

[97] Fortier LP, McKeen D, Turner K et al. The RECITE study: a Canadian prospective, multicenter study of the incidence and severity of residual neuromuscular blockade. Anesth Analg 2015; 121: 366–72.

[98] McLean DJ, Diaz-Gil D, Farhan HN et al. Dose-dependent association between intermediate-acting neuromuscular-blocking agents and postoperative respiratory complications. Anesthesiology 2015; 122: 1201–13.

[99] Savarese JJ, Miller RD, Lien CA, Caldwell JE. Pharmacology of muscle relaxants and their antagonists. Anesthesia, Churchill Livingstone, New York, 4th edition; p 417–488, 1994.

[100] Booij LH. Cyclodextrins and the emergence of sugammadex. Anaesthesia 2009; 64: 31–37.

[101] Mirakhur RK. Sugammadex in clinical practice. Anaesthesia 2009; 64: 45–54.

[102] Macario A. What does one minute of operating room time cost? J Clin Anesth. 2010; 22: 233–6.

[103] Putz L, Dransart C, Jamart J et al. Operating room discharge after deep neuromuscular block reversed with sugammadex compared to shallow block reversed with neostigmine: A randomized controlled trial. Accepted in J Clin Anesth 2016.

Section 4

# Post-hysterectomy Bowel Dysfunction

Chapter 6

# Bowel Dysfunction after Hysterectomy for Benign Conditions: Meta-Analysis and Systematic Review

Constantina Pitsillides and Hany Lashen

Additional information is available at the end of the chapter

http://dx.doi.org/10.5772/65769

**Abstract**

The aim of this study was to determine whether hysterectomy for a benign indication can cause functional gastrointestinal disorders (FGIDs). A systematic review was completed with the studies, which used a prospective design and validated quality of life questionnaires. A search strategy using Medline and Embase allowed the relevant studies published between 1950 and October 2010 to be found. Meta-analyses were also performed using the studies, which had similar research objectives. The search revealed 29 potentially suitable articles, of which 5 used a prospective design and validated quality of life questionnaires. The meta-analyses showed that the type of hysterectomy (total or subtotal) did not have an impact on whether a patient is likely to develop gastrointestinal symptoms post-surgery. The prospective studies did not show that hysterectomy for a benign indication causes FGIDs. The belief that hysterectomy can cause gastrointestinal dysfunction is based on the results of retrospective studies.

**Keywords:** gastrointestinal dysfunction, hysterectomy

## 1. Introduction

Hysterectomy is the most common gynaecological procedure that takes place [1], with approximately 100,000 being performed in the United Kingdom each year [2]. Data from 1992 showed that 20% of the women under 55 in England and Wales had a hysterectomy [3], and in 2000, 30% of women aged between 50 and 59 had the operation [4]. Over 80% of hysterectomies are performed for a benign indication [1, 3]. Symptomatic indications include menorrhagia, dysmenorrhoea and common pathologies such as uterine leiomyoma, benign ovarian process and endometriosis [1, 5].

There is controversy over whether hysterectomy can cause functional gastrointestinal disorders (FGIDs). Early reports suggested a transient change in bowel function, constipation and decreased bowel frequency [6, 7] as well as increased straining and firmer stool consistency after hysterectomy [7]. Increased anal incontinence has also been reported when bilateral salpingo-oophorectomy (BSO) was also carried out [8]. Irritable bowel syndrome (IBS) was suggested to occur de novo post-hysterectomy as many women date the onset of their symptoms to the time around their operation [9].

Functional gastrointestinal disorders (FGIDs) refer to combinations of chronic or recurrent gastrointestinal symptoms. These include irritable bowel syndrome (IBS), functional constipation, functional diarrhoea and unspecified functional bowel disorder. The female-to-male ratio for FGIDs in most categories, with the commonest being IBS and functional constipation, is 3–4:1. Symptoms are not persistent, may be intermittent, and could change from one disorder to another. Owing that FGIDs have no pathological markers [10], other methods must be used to make a diagnosis. The Rome criteria and the Manning criteria beforehand have been used to discriminate between the different FGIDs [11]. The Rome criteria, originally established by the Rome Foundation [12], have been suggested to define the FGIDs. Diagnostic guidelines have now been set for 28 adults and 17 paediatric FGIDs [13]. The guidelines are focused on five anatomical regions: oesophageal, gastroduodenal, bowel, biliary and anorectal plus an additional category of chronic abdominal pain syndrome [10].

IBS is thought to present with non-gastrointestinal features including various genitourinary and gynaecological symptoms [10] and has been frequently reported amongst women with chronic pelvic pain [14]. Chronic pelvic pain affects 33–39% of women during their lifetime and for some it is an indication for hysterectomy [15]. Further, IBS sufferers were more likely to have a hysterectomy for pain, with less noticeable improvement in symptoms. Pelvic pain typical of gynaecological origin was not more common in IBS than non-IBS sufferers [15].

When a hysterectomy is performed for benign reasons, the operation is performed mainly to improve a patient's quality of life [16], and thus, the emphasis has been placed on avoiding long-term complications. The aim of this meta-analysis is to quantitatively review the available evidence that linked hysterectomy for benign reasons to FGID. Potential sources of bias will be investigated to establish the cause of controversy in the available literature where possible.

## 2. Methods

No ethics approval was needed

### 2.1. Objectives

1. To provide an overview and a quantitative assessment of the available evidence on the effect of abdominal hysterectomy for benign disease on bowel function.

2. To eliminate the potential sources of bias in the methodology of published literature.
3. To suggest a strategy for future research.

### 2.2. Criteria for including studies for this review

A study was included if it had used a prospective design and a validated gastrointestinal quality of life questionnaire (QoLQ) or used physiological studies to assess bowel function before and after hysterectomy for benign reasons.

### 2.3. Criteria for excluding studies for this review

A study was excluded if there was a malignant indication for the hysterectomy or if a radical hysterectomy was performed. All retrospective studies and those with incomplete data at baseline and/or at follow-up were not included. The prospective studies that did not use validated QoLQs were also excluded; however, if the used questionnaire was found to be validated later on in subsequent studies, the study was included. All studies that were not published in English were excluded as suitable translators were not available.

### 2.4. Search strategy for this review

A literature search was conducted for publications between 1950 and October 2010 in Medline and Embase. The search terms used were 'hysterectomy' or 'laparoscopic hysterectomy', or 'vaginal hysterectomy'. These were cross-referenced with, 'constipation', or 'defecation', or 'bowel function', or 'faecal incontinence', or 'gastrointestinal', or 'dysfunction', or 'outcome', or 'irritable bowel syndrome', or 'functional colonic diseases', or 'gastrointestinal motility' and 'manometry', or 'anorectal', or 'anorectal physiology'.

### 2.5. Data synthesis and heterogeneity

The data included in the meta-analyses were that of three papers, which identified constipation as a possible complication of subtotal and total hysterectomy. The three papers [5, 12, 13] provided data about the number of women who suffered with constipation before and 1 year after having had the hysterectomy. The RevMan (4.2) programme was used to analyse these data. The fixed-effect model was chosen, and odds ratios and confidence intervals were calculated. Clinical heterogeneity was assessed using the $\chi^2$ and $I^2$ values.

## 3. Results

The search identified a total of 38 potential studies. Six of these used a prospective design and used validated QoLQs. One of the five studies was reported twice with one [1] and 3 years [8] of follow-up, respectively; therefore, only the 3-year follow-up study has been included in this review. Four prospective studies, which used bowel function physiological assessments both before and after the hysterectomy, were also included. **Figure 1** is a flowchart of the studies that were included and excluded from this review. **Table 1** is a summary of the prospective studies, which were included in the review, and **Table 2** shows the bowel dysfunction outcome measures and the covariates assessed in each of these studies.

The details of the excluded prospective studies are in **Table 3** [6, 9, 15, 22–25]. One of the prospective studies was published twice, one with results of the 3-year follow-up [26] and the other, the 5-year follow-up [24]. This has been included as one study. There were eight studies that were excluded as they included radical hysterectomy or patients who had the operation due to the malignant causes [27–38].

Seven retrospective studies were excluded [7, 39–45], and two studies were excluded due to not being in English, one in Dutch [46] and the other Chinese [47].

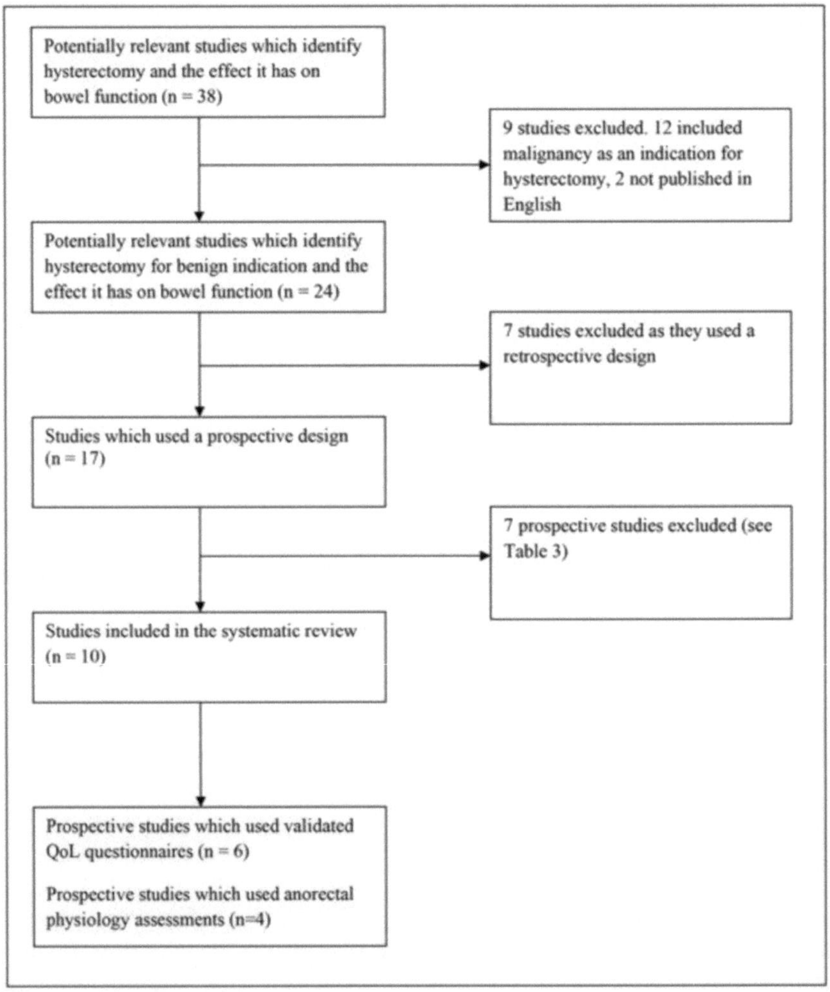


**Figure 1.** A flow chart to show the included studies.

| References | Age range of patients | Type of hysterectomy included | Study and follow-up durations | Sample size at the end of study and drop out rate | Reported outcome |
|---|---|---|---|---|---|
| Thakar et al. [5] | 29–50 SAH<br>30–59 TAH | SAH<br>TAH | 12 months<br>FU: 6 and 12 months | 240<br>119 SAH<br>121 TAH<br>14% drop out | There were no changes in bowel function at the 6- and 12-month follow-ups |
| Gimbel et al. [12] | 47.6 (mean for TAH)<br>46.6 (mean for SAH) | SAH<br>TAH | 12 months<br>FU: 12 months | 276<br>140 TAH<br>136 SAH<br>16% drop out | Hysterectomy does not cause de novo constipation in patients. TAH or SAH does not affect this outcome |
| Gimbel et al. [13] | 46.7 (mean TH)<br>48.2 (mean SH) | TAH, SAH | 12 months<br>FU: 12 months | 152<br>64 TAH<br>88 SAH<br>18% drop out | Hysterectomy does not cause de novo constipation in patients. TAH or SAH does not affect this outcome |
| Forsgren et al. [8] | 32–78 | AH<br>VH | 3 years<br>FU: 12 months, 3 years | 107<br>39 VH<br>52 AH<br>(16 BSO)<br>11% drop out | Significant increase in anal incontinence in AH patients at 1- and 3-year follow-ups. An increased risk of anal incontinence also associated with a BSO. Significant increase in defecation frequency at both follow-ups in the AH group |
| Roovers et al. [16] | 44 (mean) | TAH, SAH, VH | 3 years<br>FU: 3 years | 344<br>158 TAH<br>91 SAH<br>85 VH<br>17% drop out | SAH compared to TAH significantly increased the risk of developing constipation |
| Lashen et al. [17] | 46.5 (mean) | TAH | 12 months<br>FU: 6, 12, 24 weeks, 12 months | 95 TAH<br>31% drop out | Transient deterioration in QoL and bowel function at 6 weeks, which improved at 12 weeks, which was sustained at the additional follow-ups<br>Hysterectomy is not associated with a long-term detrimental effect on the bowel |
| Prior et al. [18] | 28–54 | VH, AH | 6 months<br>FU: 6 weeks, 6 months | 26<br>18 VH<br>8 TAH<br>0% drop out | There was a significant increase in rectal sensitivity and decreased threshold volumes required to induce sensations of gas, desire to defecate, urgency and discomfort at both follow-ups |
| Goffeng et al. [19] | 35–66 (45 mean) | SAH<br>TAH | 11–18 months | 33<br>21% drop out | Significantly lower rectal volumes before hysterectomy when compared |

| References | Age range of patients | Type of hysterectomy included | Study and follow-up durations | Sample size at the end of study and drop out rate | Reported outcome |
|---|---|---|---|---|---|
| | | | FU: 3 months, 11–18 months | | with controls. Significantly higher threshold post-hysterectomy for eliciting reflex inhibition |
| Kelly et al. [20] | 30–64 | AH<br>VH | 16 weeks<br>FU: 16 weeks | 30<br>16 AH<br>14 VH<br>0% drop out | Significant decrease in the forced voluntary contraction anal pressure in women who had more than five vaginal deliveries |
| Bharucha et al. [21] | 25–66 | VH | 12 months<br>FU: 2 months, 12 months | 19 | Post-hysterectomy no difference in anal pressures, rectal compliance and capacity compared to pre-op<br>At 12 months, there was increased rectal contractile response, but clinical significance is uncertain<br>Transient change in the desire to defecate at 2 months, which returned back to baseline (pre-hysterectomy) at 12 months<br>Reduced perception of urgency at 12 months |

TAH: total abdominal hysterectomy; SAH: subtotal abdominal hysterectomy; VH: vaginal hysterectomy; AH: abdominal hysterectomy; FU: follow-up.

**Table 1.** Characteristics of the prospective studies which used validated questionnaires or anorectal physiology.

| References | Bowel function primary or secondary | Main outcome measures | Covariates identified |
|---|---|---|---|
| Thakar et al. [5] | Secondary | Constipation, hard stools, straining to move bowels, use of laxatives, urgency, incontinence of flatus | No details were given |
| Gimbel et al. [12] | Secondary | Constipation | No details were given. |
| Gimbel et al. [13] | Secondary | Constipation | No details were given |
| Forsgren et al. [8] | Primary | Bowel-emptying difficulties, daily incomplete bowel evacuation, daily digitation and defecation frequency<br>The CCIS looked specifically at solid incontinence, liquid incontinence<br>and gas incontinence, whether the sufferer wears a pad or has had any lifestyle alterations | Parity, number vaginal deliveries, delivery of a child >4000 g, vaginal laceration at delivery, HRT after hysterectomy, BMI at surgery and at follow-up, concomitant BSO at time hysterectomy<br>Previous obstetric sphincter injury and increased age were significantly |

| References | Bowel function primary or secondary | Main outcome measures | Covariates identified |
|---|---|---|---|
| | | | associated with increased post-operative anal incontinence |
| Roovers et al. [16] | Primary | Constipation both de novo and persistent | Age, BMI, parity, history of abdominal surgery, comorbidity, menorrhagia, metrorrhagia, abdominal pain, dysmenorrhoea, fibroma present on ultrasound, maximal diameter of uterus. History of abdominal surgery significantly increased the risk of development of constipation. None of these were discovered to significantly increase the risk the persistence of constipation |
| Lashen et al. [17] | Primary | Gastrointestinal symptoms covering a range including abdominal pain, flatus, reflux, diarrhoea, constipation, dysphagia and nausea<br>A self-reported health-related QoL questionnaire was also used | Smoking and laxative use |
| Prior et al. [18] | Secondary | Maximum anal basal pressure<br>Lowest rectal volume needed to produce sensations of gas, desire to defecate, urgency of defecation, discomfort<br>Rectal compliance<br>Rectal motility index | Details from patients records were compared to the bladder urethrovesical physiology studies and not the anorectal bowel studies |
| Goffeng et al. [19] | Primary | Gastrointestinal transit time<br>Resting, anal squeeze, first sensation and urge pressures<br>Rectoanal inhibitory reflex<br>Rectal volumes | The weight of the uterus did not affect rectal volume, gastrointestinal transit time |
| Kelly et al. [20] | Primary | Mean resting pressure<br>Maximal pressure generated by forced voluntary contraction of external anal sphincter<br>Presence/absence of recto-anal inhibitory reflex<br>Rectal sensation<br>Lowest volume to produce a sensation of gas and desire to defecate | Age, this showed a significant negative correlation with mean resting anal pressure<br>More than five vaginal deliveries which caused a significant reduction in the forced voluntary contraction anal pressure |
| Bharucha et al. [21] | Primary | Anal pressures, anal squeeze and balloon expulsion<br>Rectal pressure, volume, compliance and capacity<br>Sensory thresholds for first sensation, desire to defecate and urgency | No details were given |

**Table 2.** Bowel dysfunction outcome measures (primary or secondary) and the covariates assessed in the studies included in this systematic review.

| References | Age range of patients | Type of hysterectomy included | Length study and follow-up times | Sample size at the end of study, drop out rate | Reason for exclusion/ questionnaire used | Bowel changes found |
|---|---|---|---|---|---|---|
| Longstreth et al. [15] | 43.0 (mean) | Not mentioned | 1 year<br>FU: 1 year | 164<br>5% drop out | The questionnaire used has no reference to another article and no mention of validity | IBS sufferers were more likely to have a hysterectomy due to the pain. The numbers of IBS sufferers before and after the operation were similar |
| Prior et al. [9] | 27–75 | VH<br>AH | 6 months<br>FU: 6 weeks and 12 months | 191<br>7% drop out | The questionnaire used was based on one used in a previous study. The questionnaire was pretested on patients and controls to check accuracy. No mention of validation | There was a significant decrease in non-IBS pain post-hysterectomy. There was the same number of women who had IBS before and after the hysterectomy. The majority of de novo cases were constipation predominant IBS |
| Clarke et al. [6] | <30–>55 | Not mentioned | 3 months<br>FU: 10 days, 6 weeks, 3 months | 300<br>18% drop out | Questionnaires based on evidence from published studies, on information from 35 interviews (some awaiting surgery, others having undergone hysterectomy) and on the advice of a clinician. No mention of validity tests done on the questionnaire | Significant decrease in bowel function at 10 days, with more women describing themselves as constipated. This, however, returned to pre-operative status at 6 weeks |
| Weber et al. [22] | 45.5 (mean) | TAH | 14.2 months (mean)FU: 1 year | 43<br>17% drop out | No reference was given for the questionnaire used, no mention of validation. | No significant changes with regard to frequency, straining, bloating and pain. Laxative use became a new problem in 12/23 women and was statistically significant |
| Kluivers et al. [23] | 49.9 (mean LH)<br>48.1 (mean AH) | AH<br>LH | 1 year<br>FU:<br>12 weeks,<br>1 year | 67<br>35 LH<br>32 AH<br>11% drop out | The DDI was used a Dutch validated questionnaire. The article did not give information on bowel symptoms at baseline | LH and AH did not affect bowel function at the 1-year follow-up |
| Farquhar et al. [24] | <30–45 years (lowest age not clarified) | Those who had at the conservation | 5 years<br>FU: yearly for 3 and 5 year FU | 135<br>47% drop out: 36% lost to follow-up | The questionnaire had been piloted on twenty women which had led to some changes being made. There is no | After 5 years, there were no differences in bowel symptoms before and after hysterectomy |

| References | Age range of patients | Type of hysterectomy included | Length study and follow-up times | Sample size at the end of study, drop out rate | Reason for exclusion/ questionnaire used | Bowel changes found |
|---|---|---|---|---|---|---|
| | | of at least one ovary. Not specified | | 11% as they went through the menopause and were excluded | clarification as to whether the questionnaire was validated | |
| Khoshbaten M et al. [25] | 47.14 (mean) ± 6.17 years | Not specified | 1 year FU: 3 monthly up until 1 year | 172 Implied no drop out but not explicitly written | Used a standardised questionnaire based on the Rome II criteria. No mention of validation | IBS confirmed in 8% of the hysterectomy patients at 12 months. No information is given about the symptoms at the various time points |

TAH: total abdominal hysterectomy; VH: vaginal hysterectomy; AH: abdominal hysterectomy; LH: laparoscopic hysterectomy.

**Table 3.** The excluded prospective studies which identified benign reasons for hysterectomy.

### 3.1. Studies included in the meta-analyses and heterogeneity assessment

Of the five prospective studies which used validated questionnaires, there were only three [5, 12, 13], which had similar features and allowed meta-analyses to be conducted; all used constipation as one of their main outcome measures and published data regarding constipation symptoms in women before and 1 year after total abdominal hysterectomy and subtotal abdominal hysterectomy. These can be found in **Figures 2** and **3**, respectively. A meta-analysis could not be performed on the studies, which used anorectal physiology techniques to assess bowel function [18–20] as they all used different outcome measures. There was no statistical heterogeneity amongst the studies included in the meta-analyses. An $I^2$ value for both the total and the subtotal hysterectomy was $I^2 = 0$.

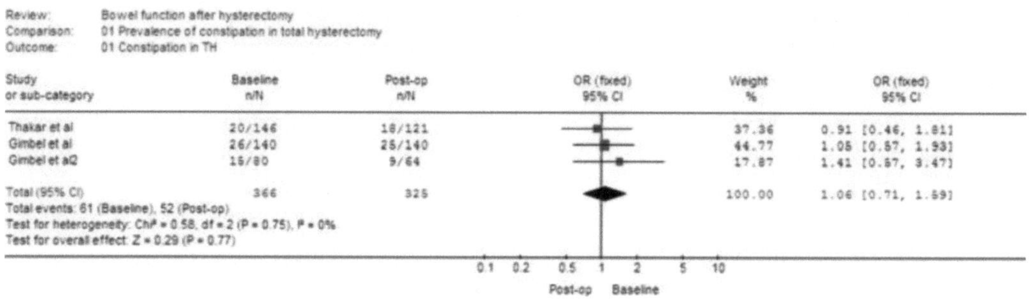


**Figure 2.** Constipation used as an indicator of bowel function before and after total hysterectomy. Gimbel et al. 2 refers to the Gimbel et al. study of 2005.

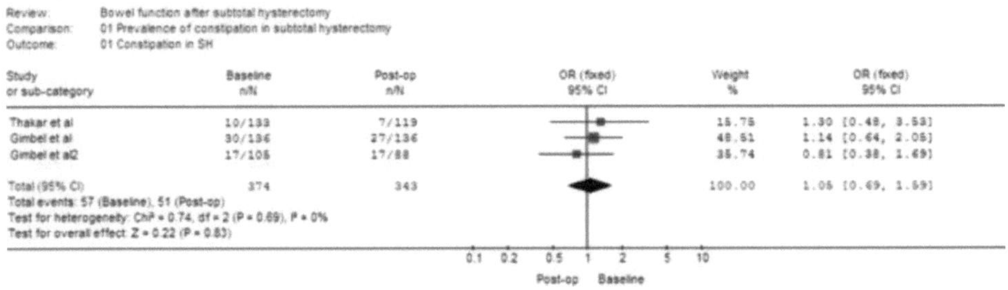


**Figure 3.** Constipation used as an indicator of bowel function before and after subtotal hysterectomy. Gimbel et al. 2 refers to the Gimbel et al. study of 2005.

### 3.2. The results of the meta-analyses

There were three studies, which were included in the meta-analyses. The odds ratios and 95% confidence intervals show that for both the total and subtotal abdominal hysterectomy, there was no statistically significant increase in the prevalence of constipation or related symptoms after a hysterectomy. The results for total abdominal hysterectomy were OR 1.06, 95% CI 0.71–1.59 (**Figure 2**) and for subtotal abdominal hysterectomy OR 1.05, 95% CI 0.69–1.59 (**Figure 3**). The studies were homogeneous, see **Figures 2** and **3**.

## 4. Discussion

Linking hysterectomy to bowel symptoms was first suggested in 1988 [41]. Several supportive retrospective studies followed, which had strong effect on the belief that hysterectomy caused bowel dysfunction. The first prospective study was published in 1990 [15]. Retrospective studies have several limitations most prominent of which is the lack of pre-operative assessment.

The earlier prospective studies were completed in 1992 by Prior et al. [9, 18]: one linking IBS and hysterectomy using a non-validated questionnaire [9] and the other used anorectal physiology techniques [18]. Longstreth et al. [15], Clarke et al. [6], Weber et al. [22] and Farquhar et al. [24] all used non-validated quality of life questionnaires and reported no association between hysterectomy and any change in bowel function. A prospective study excluded from the review [23] used validated questionnaire but offered no pre-operative bowel function assessment. Two retrospective studies used anorectal physiology reporting significant changes post-hysterectomy in one [44] but not in the other [41]. Of the retrospective studies excluded, four used validated questionnaires [7, 40, 42, 45]. They all showed bowel changes after hysterectomy. One retrospective study published used a non-validated questionnaire and reported that those who had vaginal or laparoscopic hysterectomy had a 200% increase in obstructive defecation risk [44].

Irrespective of questionnaire validation, their use has generally been criticised due to the subjective nature of such method. Further, it could be argued that using anorectal physiology tests offers objectivity; however [12] unless the patient is symptomatic, the results of such tests are of academic value which was evident in the study by Prior et al. [18]. A prospective design raises issues surrounding follow-up frequency and duration. A longer follow-up period enhances the sensitivity of symptom detection at the expense of specificity unless the symptoms can be dated back to shortly post-hysterectomy. However, a long follow may be better suited when control groups are used. When the patient is used as their own control, a long follow-up is only useful in determining the prognosis of those in whom pathology has been detected. Follow-up duration offers logistic challenges as the participants may not be contactable and their interest in the study may fade. The frequency of administering the assessment tool is important and is subject to the objectives of the study.

Increasing the frequency in the first year offers a better view of the changes in bowel function during convalescence and beyond. The design of the prospective study influences the evidence it yields. Accordingly, longitudinal cohort studies where the patient is her own control can link the operation to bowel dysfunction, while the observational controlled longitudinal studies offer mechanistic explanations.

This review has emphasised the lack of prospective studies using validated bowel function-specific QoLQ to assess bowel function after hysterectomy. The weight of evidence supports that hysterectomy does not increase the prevalence of bowel dysfunction. Of the seven suitable prospective studies which used validated questionnaires, Forsgren et al. found a significant increase in anal incontinence at 1 and 3 years [8], and Roovers et al. suggested an increased risk of constipation after subtotal compared to total hysterectomy [16]. Lashen et al. used three validated QoL questionnaires to provide a holistic assessment of the patients' QoL as well as their bowel symptoms. A transient worsening of bowel symptoms was noted at the 6-week follow-up, but this resolved by 12 weeks and there was no further deterioration noted at subsequent follow-ups [17]. The anorectal physiology studies were conflicting: two studies reporting significant changes after hysterectomy [18, 19] one reported changes only in the women who had more than five vaginal deliveries, [20] and the other found only subtle effects on anorectal sensorimotor functions [21].

Thakar et al. used a randomized double-blind trial to compare the effects of total abdominal hysterectomy (TAH) and subtotal abdominal hysterectomy (SAH). They reported no post-operative change in bowel function irrespective of the method used or other operative variables [5]. The questionnaire they used was referenced to previous work [40] that referred to an earlier study [48], finally leading to an article that was published in 1978 [49]. Although the questionnaire was validated at some point, it was designed before the Rome II criteria were established. Other studies used the same questionnaire [12, 13]. Gimbel et al. (2003) randomised patients into TAH and SAH and reported no significant increase in constipation irrespective of the type of hysterectomy [12, 13]. However, there was a non-significant decrease in constipation reporting among SAH patients (20% pre-operatively to 14% post-operatively).

Others reported increased anal incontinence at 1 and 3 year after TAH [8]. Further, a significant increase in anal incontinence was also reported with concomitant BSO at 1 year, but the numbers decreased by the third year. The vaginal hysterectomy group had an increase in anal incontinence at 3 years only, but no complete incontinence. Analysing the patients' demographic data revealed that previous obstetric sphincter injury and increased age were associated with the observed increased risk of post-hysterectomy anal incontinence [8]. They published the 1-year follow-up of the same study separately [1], and this was not included in the meta-analysis. They used two questionnaires: the first had been developed by the Swedish Society of Colorectal Surgeons and the second used an index based on the Cleveland Clinic Incontinence Score, which measured the severity of faecal incontinence using an analogue scale [8].

Roovers et al. used strict definition criteria to investigate the development of de novo post-hysterectomy constipation that persisted for the duration of the study's follow-up period. At the 3-year mark, only 2% of the TAH patients developed de novo constipation, while those who had SAH reported a higher rate of constipation which persisted in half the patients who reported pre-operative constipation [16]. The Defecation Distress Inventory (DDI) was collaborated after studying the literature and international definitions, interviewing sufferers of constipation and faecal incontinence and by interviewing three specialists in surgery, and obstetrics and gynaecology.

The anorectal physiology studies were also of importance in this systematic review. Some studies assessed the patients' symptoms [18, 19, 21]. Prior et al. revealed significant changes in the anorectal physiology tests, but did not uncover any changes in gastrointestinal symptoms [18]. Goffeng et al. used interviews and uncovered some significant findings, for example, a decrease in abdominal pain and dyspareunia post-operatively, but were not associated with any changes discovered in the physiology tests [19]. Constipation was not assessed using a specific definition, but was dependent on the participant's subjective recollection. It is imperative to clarify that although gaining an insight into patients' symptoms is important, there was no indication in either study to the validity of the methods used to gain these data.

Kelly et al. did not detect any changes in the mean resting anal pressure after hysterectomy, but forced voluntary contraction anal pressure was significantly lower at 4-month post-operatively. They assigned that to having more than five vaginal births. The mean forced voluntary contraction pressure was significantly lower in these women compared to those who had undergone <5 deliveries. The number of deliveries did not affect the mean resting or maximal forced voluntary contraction pressures. Other physiology tests were not affected by hysterectomy [20]. Bharucha found increased rectal stiffness at 12 months post-hysterectomy, but its significance was uncertain and a reduced perception of rectal urgency at 12 months, which was not statistically significant. A validated bowel symptoms questionnaire was used, but there are not much data published as to the results of the questionnaire [21]. All the anorectal physiology studies [18–20] had small numbers of participants, ranging from 19 to 33 which is under representative of the population. The numbers are small, which could indicate a lack of representation.

Goffeng et al. used interviews as well as the anorectal physiology methods comparing the patients to themselves and a control group. No significant differences were observed for the resting and anal squeeze pressures when hysterectomy patients were compared with the controls, and when pre-operative and post-operative findings were compared. Rectal volumes were significantly lower in the hysterectomy patients before and after the operation compared to controls and were not influenced by the uterine weight. Higher thresholds for provoking reflex inhibition were reported in hysterectomy patients post-operatively. There were no significant changes in gastrointestinal transit time or between the total and subtotal hysterectomy group findings [19].

Gimbel et al. [12] and Thakar et al. [5] randomised the women in their studies to total or subtotal abdominal hysterectomy, thus allowing the comparison of the outcomes of the two procedures [5, 12]. It was argued that the lack of blinding and non-randomisation was likely to overestimate the intervention effect, in this case the type of hysterectomy [12].

Roovers et al. and Forsgren et al. had the longest follow-up of 3 years [8, 16]; however, Roovers et al. did not address the ovary status; therefore, it is difficult to verify if oophorectomy had any effect on the risk of incontinence as reported by Forsgren et al. Both studies analysed the impact of patients' demography on the studies' outcomes, which lacked in previous work [5, 12, 13]

The findings of the study by Forsgren et al. were unique in that it was the first study to identify a relationship between hysterectomy and anal incontinence. There are no obvious reasons or underlying mechanisms; however, the type of questionnaire used may explain their findings; until their findings are verified, they should be interpreted with caution [8]. The validity of the questionnaire used by Thakar et al. is also in question as it was developed after the Rome II criteria [5].

The meta-analyses findings used Forrest plots to identify whether constipation was likely to occur after hysterectomy in subtotal and total abdominal hysterectomy. It was evident that the prevalence of constipation did not change post-operatively indicating that hysterectomy did not increase the risk of constipation as previously suggested. Further, the three studies [5, 12, 13] that were included in this meta-analysis comprised more than 300 patients, which is bigger than any individual prospective studies, thus providing a reliable evidence.

Seven prospective studies were excluded for not using validated questionnaires in six studies [6, 15, 18, 22, 24, 25], and the sixth was excluded as they [23] did not give any pre-operative details about bowel function despite using a validated questionnaire (the DDI). Using a validated questionnaire is essential for this type of studies so that the predictive value and reproducibility of the research tools are known; otherwise, the methodology would be flawed. The details of the excluded studies are given in **Table 3**.

All post-radical hysterectomy studies and those in which hysterectomy was carried out for malignancy totalling 12 studies were excluded. Of these studies, six used a prospective design [28, 29, 33, 34, 36, 38] and one used anorectal physiology techniques to assess reporting positive findings after the operation [29]. Barnes et al. also included anorectal physiology techniques and found post-operative changes in all their participants [33]. Pieterse et al. reported that radiotherapy did not affect colorectal motility and that radical hysterectomy had a negative impact on diarrhoea symptoms when compared to controls [27]. The study by Guthrie et al. made conclusions based on the hysterectomy group as a whole. They did not discuss the hysterectomy group who had the operation performed for malignancy separately from those who had the procedure for a benign indication [34]. Veirhout et al. described two case reports of patients who suffered with severe slow-transit constipation that responded only to left-sided hemicolectomy [32]. Three of the studies used a retrospective design and found that radical hysterectomy induced bowel problems including constipation [28, 31], defecation problems [30], prolonged straining and increased use of laxatives [31].

The rationale for excluding such studies was that radical surgery is likely to be associated with a higher risk of damage to surrounding nerves and pelvic floor. Nerve sparing techniques used with radical hysterectomy have been found to significantly improve morbidity post-op compared to those who had no nerve sparing [35, 36]. Further, those who had a malignancy may also receive adjuvant radiotherapy therapy, which can affect the bowel function and pelvic vasculature. Moreover, there is consistent evidence indicating that cancer along with its therapy and the uncertain future pertinent to it are associated with depression and anxiety potentially leading to psychological problems, which can persist even after successful treatment [50]. These factors in turn are likely to impact on the bowel function [51].

Due to the small numbers of studies that were available for this meta-analysis, it was not possible to produce a funnel plot to assess the publication bias. However, the publication bias is generally speaking inevitable as the studies reporting positive findings are more likely to hit the press. Further, there was evident homogeneity in the included studies supporting the overall effect.

## 5. Conclusion

Overall, the controversy over whether hysterectomy causes bowel dysfunction stems mainly from the retrospective studies. The weight of evidence in the prospective studies favours that hysterectomy has no effect on bowel function; however, the physiological studies suggest post-operative changes that are not enough to cause symptoms. Future research should incorporate different designs and incorporate both symptomatic assessment using disease-/organ-specific QoL questionnaires and anorectal physiology, so that a global view could be obtained.

### Abbreviations

| | |
|---|---|
| AH | Abdominal hysterectomy |
| FU | Follow-up |
| QoLQ | Quality of life questionnaire |
| SAH | Subtotal abdominal hysterectomy |
| TAH | Total abdominal hysterectomy |
| VH | Vaginal hysterectomy |

## Author details

Constantina Pitsillides and Hany Lashen*

*Address all correspondence to: h.lashen@sheffield.ac.uk

University of Sheffield and Sheffield Teaching Hospitals NHS Foundation Trust, Sheffield, UK

## References

[1] Altman D, Zetterström J, Lopez A, Pollack J, Nordenstam J, Mellgren A. Effect of hysterectomy on bowel function. Diseases of the Colon & Rectum. 2004;47:502–509. doi: 10.1007/s10350-003-0087-5

[2] Clayton RD. Hysterectomy. Best Practice & Research in Clinical Obstetrics & Gynaecology. 2006;20:73–87. doi:10.1016/j.bpobgyn.2005.09.007

[3] Vessey MP, Villard-Mackintosh L, McPherson K, Coulter A, Yeates D. The epidemiology of hysterectomy: findings in a large cohort study. British Journal of Obstetrics & Gynaecology. 1992;99:402–407. doi:10.1111/j.1471-0528.1992.tb13758.x

[4] Kennedy TM, Jones RH. The epidemiology of hysterectomy and irritable bowel syndrome in a UK population. International Journal of Clinical Practice. 2000;54:647–650.

[5] Thakar R, Ayers S, Clarkson P, Stanton S, Manyonda I. Outcomes after total versus subtotal abdominal hysterectomy. New England Journal of Medicine. 2002;347:1318–1325. doi:10.1056/NEJMoa013336

[6] Clarke A, Black N, Rowe P, Mott S, Howle K. Indications for and outcome of total abdominal hysterectomy for benign disease: a prospective cohort study. British Journal of Obstetrics & Gynaecology. 1995;102:611–620. doi:10.1111/j.1471-0528.1995.tb11398.x

[7] Taylor T, Smith AN, Fulton M. Effects of hysterectomy on bowel and bladder function. International Journal of Colorectal Disease. 1990;5(4):228–231. doi:10.1007/BF00303282

[8] Forsgren C, Zetterström J, Lopez A, Nordenstam J, Anzen B, Altman D. Effects of hysterectomy on bowel function: a three-year, prospective cohort study. Diseases of the Colon & Rectum. 2007;50(8):1139–1145.

[9] Prior A, Stanley KM, Smith AR, Read NW. Relation between hysterectomy and the irritable bowel: a prospective study. Gut. 1992;33:814–817. doi:10.1136/gut.33.6.814

[10] Whorwell PJ, McCallum M, Creed FH, Roberts CT. Non-colonic features of irritable bowel syndrome. Gut. 1986;27:37–40. doi:10.1136/gut.27.1.37

[11] Corrazziari E. Definition and epidemiology of functional gastrointestinal disorders. Best Practice & Research in Clinical Gastroenterology. 2004;18:613–631. doi:10.1016/j.bpg.2004.04.012

[12] Gimbel H, Zobbe V, Andersen BM, Filtenborg T, Gluud C, Tabor A. Randomised controlled trial of total compared with subtotal hysterectomy with one-year follow up results. BJOG: An International Journal of Obstetrics & Gynaecology. 2003;110:1088–1098. doi:10.1111/j.1471-0528.2003.02395.x

[13] Gimbel H, Zobbe V, Andersen BM, Gluud C, Ottesen BS, Tabor A, Danish Hysterectomy Group. Total versus subtotal hysterectomy: an observational study with one-year follow-up. Australian & New Zealand Journal of Obstetrics & Gynaecology. 2005;45:64–67. doi:10.1111/j.1479-828X.2005.00350.x

[14] Zondervan KT, Yudkin PL, Vessey MP, Jenkinson CP, Dawes MG, Barlow DH, Kennedy SH. Chronic pelvic pain in the community—symptoms, investigations, and diagnoses. American Journal of Obstetrics & Gynecology. 2001;184:1149–1155. doi:10.1067/mob.2001.112904

[15] Longstreth GF, Preskill DB, Youkeles L. Irritable bowel syndrome in women having diagnostic laparoscopy or hysterectomy. Relation to gynecologic features and outcome. Digestive Diseases & Sciences. 1990;35:1285–1290. doi:10.1007/BF01536421

[16] Roovers JP, van der Bom JG, van der Vaart CH, Hys VA Study Group. Hysterectomy does not cause constipation. Diseases of the Colon & Rectum. 2008;51:1068–1072. doi:10.1007/s10350-007-9147-6

[17] Lashen H, Jones GL, Durua C, Pitsillides C, Radley S, Jacquesb RM, McAlindon M. Bowel dysfunction after total abdominal hysterectomy for benign conditions: a prospective longitudinal study. European Journal of Gastroenterology & Hepatology. 2013;25:1217–1222. doi:10.1097/MEG.0b013e328362dc5e

[18] Prior A, Stanley K, Smith AR, Read NW. Effect of hysterectomy on anorectal and urethrovesical physiology. Gut. 1992;33:264–267. doi:10.1136/gut.33.2.264

[19] Goffeng AR, Andersch B, Antov S, Berndtsson I, Oresland T, Hulten L. Does simple hysterectomy alter bowel function? Annales Chirurgiae et Gynaecologiae. 1997;86:298–303.

[20] Kelly JL, O'Riordain DS, Jones E, Alawi E, O'Riordain MG, Kirwan WO. The effect of hysterectomy on ano-rectal physiology. International Journal of Colorectal Disease. 1998;13:116–118. doi:10.1007/s003840050147

[21] Bharucha AE, Klingele CJ, Gebhart JB, Zinsmeister AR. Effects of vaginal hysterectomy on anorectal sensorimotor functions—a prospective study. Neurogastroenterology Motility. 2012;24:235–241. doi:10.1111/j.1365-2982.2011.01825.x

[22] Weber AM, Walters MD, Schover LR, Church JM, Piedmonte MR. Functional outcomes and satisfaction after abdominal hysterectomy. American Journal of Obstetrics & Gynecology. 1999;181:530–535. doi:10.1016/S0002-9378(99)70488-6

[23] Kluivers KB, Mol BW, Bremer GL, Brölmann HA, Vierhout ME, Bongers MY. Pelvic organ function in randomized patients undergoing laparoscopic or abdominal hysterectomy. Journal of Minimally Invasive Gynecology. 2007;14:442–448. doi:10.1016/j.jmig.2007.02.015

[24] Farquhar CM, Sadler L, Stewart AW. A prospective study of outcome five years after hysterectomy in premenopausal women. Australian & New Zealand Journal of Obstetrics & Gynaecology. 2008;48:510–516. doi:10.1111/j.1479-828X.2008.00893.x

[25] Khoshbaten M, Melli MS, Fattahi MJ, Sharifi N, Mostafavi SA, Pourhoseingholi MA. Irritable bowel syndrome in women undergoing hysterectomy and tubular ligation. Gastroenterology and Hepatology from Bed to Bench. 2011;4:138–141.

[26] Farquhar CM, Harvey SA, Yu Y, Sadler L, Stewart AW. A prospective study of 3 years of outcomes after hysterectomy with and without oophorectomy. American Journal of Obstetrics and Gynecology. 2006;194:711–717. doi:10.1016/j.ajog.2005.08.066

[27] Pieterse QD, Maas CP, ter Kuile MM, Lowik M, van Eijkeren MA, Trimbos JB, Kenter GG. An observational longitudinal study to evaluate miction, defecation, and sexual function after radical hysterectomy with pelvic lymphadenectomy for early-stage cervical cancer. International Journal of Gynecological Cancer. 2006;16:1119–1129. doi:10.1111/j.1525-1438.2006.00461.x

[28] Choi JS, Myung SJ, Byeon JS, Park WC, Kim KJ, Yang SK, Yoon IJ, Kwon OR, Ko JE, Hong WS, Kim JH, Min YI. Clinical characteristics of patients with chronic constipation after radical hysterectomy or delivery. Korean Journal of Gastroenterology. 2004;44:267–274.

[29] Sood AK, Nygaard I, Shahin MS, Sorosky JI, Lutgendorf SK, Rao SS. Anorectal dysfunction after surgical treatment for cervical cancer. Journal of the American College of Surgeons. 2002;195:513–519. doi:10.1016/S1072-7515(02)01311-X

[30] van Dam JH, Gosseling MJ, Drogendijk AC, Hop WC, Schouten WR. Changes in bowel function after hysterectomy. Diseases of the Colon & Rectum. 1997;40:1342–1347. doi:10.1007/BF02050820

[31] Schreuder HW, Vierhout ME, Veen HF. Disabling constipation following Wertheim's radical hysterectomy. Nederlands Tijdschrift voor Geneeskunde. 1993;137:1059–1062.

[32] Vierhout ME, Schreuder HW, Veen HF. Severe slow-transit constipation following radical hysterectomy. Gynecologic Oncology. 1993;51:401–403. doi:10.1006/gyno.1993.1311

[33] Barnes W, Waggoner S, Delgado G, Maher K, Potkul R, Barter J, Benjamin S. Manometric characterization of rectal dysfunction following radical hysterectomy. Gynecologic Oncology. 1991;42:116–119. doi:10.1016/0090-8258(91)90329-4

[34] Guthrie JR, Clark MS, Dennerstein L. A prospective study of outcomes after hysterectomy in mid-aged Australian-born women. Climacteric. 2007;10:171–177. doi: 10.1080/13697130601170018

[35] Ceccaroni M, Roviglione G, Spagnolo E, Casadio P, Clarizia R, Peiretti M, Bruni F, Peters I, Aletti G. Pelvic dysfunctions and quality of life after nerve-sparing radical hysterectomy: a multicenter comparative study. Anticancer Research. 2012;32:581–588.

[36] Cibula D, Velechovska P, Slama J, Fischerova D, Pinkavova I, Pavlista D, Dundr P, Hill M, Freitag P, Zikan M. Late morbidity following nerve-sparing radical hysterectomy. Gynecologic Oncology. 2010;116:506–511. doi:10.1016/j.ygyno.2009.10.061

[37] Park SK, Myung SJ, Jung KW, Chun YH, Yang DH, Seo SY, Ku HS, Yoon IJ, Kim KJ, Ye BD, Byeon JS, Jung HY, Yang SK, Kim JH. Biofeedback therapy for female patients with constipation caused by radical hysterectomy or vaginal delivery. Journal of Gastroenterology & Hepatology. 2013;28:1133–1140. doi:10.1111/jgh.12158

[38] Pieterse QD, Kenter G, Maas CP, de Kroon CD, Creutzberg CL, Trimbos JB, Ter Kuile MM. Self-reported sexual, bowel and bladder function in cervical cancer patients following different treatment modalities: longitudinal prospective cohort study. International Journal of Gynaecological Cancer. 2013;23:1717–1725. doi:10.1097/IGC.0b013e3182a80a65

[39] Gaj F, Trecca A, Scozzafava U, Talarico C, Caviglia R, Scardamaglia F, Parisi CM, Carboni M. Constipation following hysterectomy. Retrospective study based on 105 cases. Minerva Ginecologica. 1995;47:83–87.

[40] Heaton KW, Parker D, Cripps H. Bowel function and irritable bowel symptoms after hysterectomy and cholecystectomy—a population based study. Gut. 1993;34:1108–1111. doi:10.1136/gut.34.8.1108

[41] Roe AM, Bartolo DC, Mortensen NJ. Slow transit constipation. Comparison between patients with or without previous hysterectomy. Digestive Diseases & Sciences. 1988;33:1159–1163. doi:10.1007/BF01535794

[42] Roovers JP, van der Bom JG, Huub van der Vaart C, Fousert DM, Heintz AP. Does mode of hysterectomy influence micturition and defecation? Acta Obstetricia et Gynecologica Scandinavica. 2001;80:945–951. doi:10.1034/j.1600-0412.2001.801012.x

[43] Smith AN, Varma JS, Binnie NR, Papachrysostomou M. Disordered colorectal motility in intractable constipation following hysterectomy. British Journal of Surgery. 1990;77:1361–1365. doi:10.1002/bjs.1800771214

[44] Varma MG, Hart SL, Brown JS, Creasman J, Van Den Eeden SK, Thom DH. Obstructive defecation in middle-aged women. Digestive Diseases & Sciences 2008;53:2702–2709. doi:10.1007/s10620-008-0226-x

[45] Smith TM, Menees SB, Xu X, Saad RJ, Chey WD, Fenner DE. Factors associated with quality of life among women with fecal incontinence. International Urogynecology Journal. 2013;24:493–499. doi:10.1007/s00192-012-1889-6

[46] Roovers JP, Weenen M, van der Bom JG, van der Vaart CH. Defecation complaints after hysterectomy because of a benign condition are rare; a prospective study. Nederlands Tijdschrift voor Geneeskunde. 2007;151:1239–1243.

[47] Miao YL, Zhou R, Wang JL. Survey of long term female pelvic floor function and sexual life status after total hysterectomy. Zhonghua fu Chan ke za zhi. 2012;47:496–499.

[48] Heaton KW, O'Donnell LJ, Braddon FE, Mountford RA, Hughes AO, Cripps PJ. Symptoms of irritable bowel syndrome in a British urban community: consulters and nonconsulters. Gastroenterology. 1992;102:1962–1967.

[49] Manning AP, Thompson WG, Heaton KW, Morris AF. Towards positive diagnosis of the irritable bowel. British Medical Journal. 1978;2:653–654. doi:10.1136/bmj.2.6138.653

[50] Cooper R, Mishra G, Hardy R, Kuh D. Hysterectomy and subsequent psychological health: findings from a British birth cohort study. Journal of Affective Disorders. 2009;115:122–130. doi:10.1016/j.jad.2008.08.017

[51] Quigley EM. Current concepts of the irritable bowel syndrome. Scandinavian Journal of Gastroenterology Supplement. 2003;237:1–8. doi:10.1080/00855910310001403